D1229326

"LISTEN TO ME, I AM STILL SOMEBODY"

UNDERSTANDING THE ALZHEIMER'S DISEASE SUFFERER

SANDRA M. KEHOE, RN

Bill & Kathy
Hope my book
helps you "understand"
Sandy
3/16/08

Universal Publishers
Boca Raton, Florida

"Listen to Me, I'm Still Somebody":
Understanding the Alzheimer's Disease Sufferer

Copyright © 2008 Sandra M. Kehoe
All rights reserved.

Universal Publishers
Boca Raton, Florida • USA
2008

ISBN-10: 1-58112- 988-2
ISBN-13: 978-1-58112-988-5

www.universal-publishers.com

ACKNOWLEDGMENTS

This book is the culmination of 25 years of caring for and learning from all the professionals in Alzheimer's disease research and education and the sufferers of this dreaded disease and their families.

It could not have been accomplished without the loving friendship of my colleagues, Brenda Carr and Fran Floersheimer who have remained with the Alzheimer's Association, Houston and Southeast Texas Chapter. With their support and our collective expertise, the work of learning about the special needs of the Alzheimer's Disease sufferer and their families was begun.

We simply studied the needs of the Alzheimer's Disease sufferer by observing their behaviors and discussing the difficulties encountered by the families taking care of them. The knowledge gained enabled us to design environments and plans of care that would assure the best quality of life. We listened and we learned.

We were hoping as a group that these special environments would spread throughout all areas of care, since actually it is patient oriented care. This in itself was a leap of faith since traditionally, at that time, we "the medical community" would create the environment that we decided was the best one and attempt to put people in it without truly understanding their special needs. We were trying to put square pegs in round holes.

Ultimately this collective knowledge was used in developing comprehensive workshops to train professionals and help family care givers create these specialized living environments. This knowledge has helped the Long Term Care Industry, Assisted Living Industry, Day Care Industry and families create these Alzheimer's friendly areas. They now understand that these areas are not purely structural in nature. Understanding the nuances of the disease process is necessary to successfully manage the behaviors of the person with Alzheimer's Disease.

Armed with this knowledge and the help of community professionals, the Alzheimer's Disease sufferer can be managed at home for a longer period of time, if the family dynamics permit.

This book has been a dream of mine for several years. I must thank my family and friends for their encouragement and my dear friend and fellow Rotarian, Bill Sikes, for his countless hours of computer work in helping me make my dream a reality.

Sandy

PROLOGUE

I have been fortunate to receive very positive reaction to my lectures. I seem to be able to put the information about the Alzheimer's Disease process and its effects on the sufferers and their families in a very understandable, personal way. These occasions are as meaningful to me as they are to the participants. I know that what they learn from me will be used to help themselves and others survive the life-shattering effects of this disease.

This book is my attempt to put the information I present during my lectures and workshops in written form. I am attempting to write it in a conversational way. I want those who read my book to *hear* me.

Instead of talking to a group, I found myself talking to my computer. A strange thing happened to me, though; I was crying. It seemed that all of the times I had maintained my composure, while the many families I met told me of the horrors they were experiencing, had a lasting effect. Apparently that composure was not needed when I was alone with my computer. This reaction surprised me.

Mercifully, I have had no one in my family suffer with this disease. I was introduced to this devastating disease in 1983. We had moved to Texas and I was working in a nursing home as a Community Relation Representative. The Nursing home, along with several in the area, was attempting to develop Alzheimer's and Related Dementia units. I knew very little about this disease, so I contacted the Alzheimer's Association to find out about any workshops that were available in the community. I read all that I could find about this strange disease, and I also attended family support groups. I would sit there and listen in awe to the families talk about the frightening things that have happened to their families because of this disease. They were desperate for any information and support they could find to help them survive this nightmare.

The pain and sadness expressed by the care givers at these meetings left a lasting impression on me. I knew at that time that I must do something, anything, to help ease this pain. I learned as much as I could and began to volunteer with the Alzheimer's Assoc. in Houston. I joined with other professionals and began lecturing, facilitating support groups and setting up workshops for other professionals and helping facilities like ours to set up specialized environments.

One would expect that the staffs of competitor facilities and companies would find it difficult to work together. We didn't. The needs of the Alzheimer's Disease sufferers and their families brought us together for a greater purpose. We became the members of the Advisory committee, Education Committee and the Family Support Committee of our local chapter. This time was the most amazing time in my life and was the best example of what a group of like-minded individuals can do when they combine their expertise to benefit the community.

Actually, I learned that this is how the National Alzheimer's and Related Dementia Association came to be in the first place. Families were desperate for information, as this disease was becoming more visible. Alzheimer's Disease had been around for years as a no-named mental and physical deterioration that was not spoken about in polite society. It was seen as a mental illness and families kept its existence a secret due to the social disgrace it implied. It was a few brave families that sought out other families suffering with this disease in an attempt to disseminate the few bits of information they had and offer support. They would take donations during these meetings in order to get the money to mail out the meeting notices and information to any and all families who needed it.

If anyone doubts that a small group of people can move mountains, just remember this. These very families, meeting for support and information, began meeting all over the country. These were the beginnings of The National Alzheimer's and Related Disease Association we know today. Impressive, huh?

I hope the readers of this book can feel the love and concern I have for the Alzheimer's Disease sufferer and their families and for professionals who are gathering information in order to relieve some of the sadness and suffering associated with this disease process. I humbly pray that my book will bring some peace to the families and encouragement to these professionals.

Sandy

DEDICATION

This book is dedicated to my son, Mike, who inspired me to pursue the education that has allowed me to help so many Alzheimer's Disease sufferers and their families.

FOREWORD

I will begin this book as I do my lectures, with a poem. I believe that hearing, or in this case reading, this poem prepares the participant for and makes them receptive to the information about caring for the Alzheimer's Disease sufferer.

I have had this poem for the last twenty five years. It was relevant then and it is relevant today. As I understand it, the poem was written by a Alzheimer's Disease sufferer who lived in California.

ADVICE ON CARING FOR ALZHEIMER PATIENTS

By
Joy Glenner
San Diego, CA

Dear family and friends:
Please try to understand
What I am now, not think of me
As I was.
I am alone, shut in
With my fears,
My frustration,
My forgetfulness.
Forgive me if I strike out at you.
Why do I do that?
What has happened to me?
I cannot cope with this alien world.
I feel threatened. I am frightened.
Speak softly, approach slowly.
Repeat again and again what you want of me.
Those twisted tangles in my brain
Have messed up my world.
Be patient, for I do love you,
And I need your help and love
So very , very much.
Your Alzheimer Patient.

CONTENTS

1

MEMORY LOSS
It is not always Alzheimer's Disease

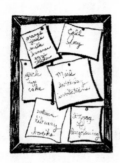

Educating the community about the Alzheimer's Disease process and the specialized treatment required has been the most rewarding aspect of my professional career.

My colleagues and I have worked tirelessly for years to educate the community, so the Alzheimer's Disease sufferers and their families would be able to receive more help.

With the help of increased visibility in the media and the disclosure that our late president Ronald Reagan suffered from this dreaded disease, Alzheimer's Disease is more clearly understood. Funding for care and research has increased significantly.

So, apparently, has the fear of having the disease. An understandable reaction, but one we did not foresee. We did not realize all this information was creating a significant amount of fear along with the increased awareness. We all see the warning signs in publications on tv and on the internet frequently. Articles about Alzheimer's Disease appear everywhere as well.

Although Alzheimer's Disease is the most common dementia, it is not the only reason for the symptoms experienced. Many medical conditions with similar symptoms are now going undiagnosed.

The community is now afraid to tell anyone, including their physicians, that they are experiencing these symptoms for fear the reason might be Alzheimer's Disease.

Confusion and memory loss can have many causes. Alzheimer's Disease is only one reason for this type of condition. That is why a proper examination and interview and family history are so vital. Many conditions and illnesses can have memory loss and confusion as one of their symptoms.

We'll begin with a few simple explanations.

Stress:

Any interference that disturbs a person's healthy mental and physical well-being. Continued exposure to stress often leads to mental and physical symptoms such as anxiety and depression. Stress can also cause memory loss.

We will refer to this type of stress induced memory loss as lapses. We all have lapses. Haven't you ever walked into a room and forgotten why you were there? Be Honest Now!

A professor of psychology was discussing the possibility of lapses in our every day stressful lives. There was one student who raised his hand to proclaim that he never has lapses. He claimed to be in complete control of his mental faculties at all times. Isn't there always one in the group?

The professor congratulated him on his ability. He requested that the student do a test to reinforce his unusual ability and asked that he share the results with the class when they next met. The student was to keep a record of each time he entered a room and forgot why he was there, each time he misplaced his keys, glasses, his car in a large parking lot, when he finds the sugar in the refrigerator, arrived late for an appointment or forgot the appointment all together. The student assured the professor these things never happen to him. The professor asked the student to please humor him and try the test anyway.

The next time the class met, the professor asked the student to share the results of the exercise with the class. The student had three pages of lapses he had experienced.

I might add that this particular student was very attentive for the remainder of the discussion on stress and how it affects our lives. That's one for all the teachers out there.

Delirium:

An acute state of confusion in which the activity of the brain is affected by fever, drugs, poisons or injury. The elderly are particularly prone to acute confusional states from certain drugs, such as barbiturates, tranquilizers or alcohol. Many older persons can have delirium after surgery, due to the mixture of sedatives, anesthesia and pain relievers. This delirium can take several days or even weeks to clear.

Confusion:

A disorganized mental state in which the abilities to remember, think clearly and reason are impaired. Confusion does not always indicate dementia.

Many disorders can cause dementia-like symptoms:

Medication reactions:

Many medications can have side effects that mimic the symptoms of dementia.

While presenting a workshop on handling medication with a group of seniors who were attending a day center, one of the participants told me she puts all of her medications in a bowl in her dining room and takes a handful once a day. I really thought she was joking; unfortunately, she wasn't.

Although her behavior is not common, many people do not take medications seriously. Most often they mix their prescribed medications with over the counter purchases. They have a tendency to share their medications with others. Not realizing that their friend's reaction to their medication can be very different.

Many people also have a tendency to keep medications after their expiration date, as well. I was discussing medication reactions with a group of health care professionals, which luckily included a Pharmacist. I asked him, as an example to the group, if he could assure us that medications that have expired have the same chemical structure. He said he could not.

Most people also assume all of their doctors know all the medications they are taking. They don't! The best thing to do is take a list of all the medications that you are taking, including the over the counter medication you have prescribed for yourself, to each physician you visit. The reaction of many of these medications can be the very reason you felt bad enough to make the appointment with your physician in the first place.

Dehydration:

Older persons dehydrate more rapidly. We all have an indicator in our brains that trigger our thirst when we need water. In the elderly, this trigger slows down. You can see how this can be a severe problem for the Alzheimer's disease sufferer. Not only is their natural alert system not working, their ability to recognize the problem and initiate the drinking of a glass of water is diminished as well.

When we do not get enough water the chemicals in our body concentrate and cause symptoms similar to those caused by dementia. Interestingly, taking too much water can dilute these same chemicals and cause just as serious a reaction.

Hypoglycemia:

Not having enough sugar in the blood stream can cause confusion and personality changes. It is not un-common for a diabetic who is experiencing low blood sugar to initially be accused of being inebriated be-cause of their reaction to low blood sugar.

Hypothyroid Disease:

An underactive thyroid can cause confusion, mem-ory loss and personality changes. When discovered, the treatment is to replace the thyroxin that has been diminished by the disorder. The symptoms gradually disappear.

Anemia:

Chronic alcoholism can deplete vitamin B-1, which can severely impair mental abilities. Severe deficiencies in vitamin B-6 can lead to a neurological illness with features of dementia. Pernicious anemia, an impaired ability to absorb vitamin B-12, can also cause personality changes. The symptoms of confusion, memory loss and weakness disappear with treatment.

Urinary Tract Infection:

Especially devastating in the elderly. It may have manifestations that are hard to identify. Classically one experiences burning, spasms, foul odor of the urine, an elevated temperature and sometimes, in a severe urinary tract infection, blood may appear in the urine. However, the symptoms can be disguised, as they were in an elderly man I cared for. The only indication that he had a urinary tract infection was when he suddenly fell forward while walking across the room. A large gash on his forehead and an emergency trip to the hospital clarified his sudden loss of balance as a very severe urinary tract infection.

Depression:

Confusion, apathy and forgetfulness are associated with depression and sometimes mistaken for dementia, especially in the elderly.

Many years ago, I had the privilege of meeting a physician in Houston who was in the process of researching depression. Again, one of the times I was honored to be in the presence of an incredible professional who allowed me to see this Alzheimer's Disease process so clearly.

He shared with me his concern that so many times, too many times, the symptoms of depression can mimic the aspects of Alzheimer's Disease. This includes confusion, memory loss, personality changes, reclusive behavior, mood swings and the loss of the ability to continue one's personal care. If diagnosed early and the needed medication, started the person will begin to recover, usually in about four to six weeks. If left undiagnosed, the person will sink deeper into the depression, never to recover. It is usually in the elderly that the symptoms of depression go undiagnosed more frequently.

Sadly, we as a society had a tendency to believe an elderly person showing up at the emergency room in a confused state was to be expected. This situation might not have alarmed the staff several years ago. Luckily we have improved our knowledge of elder care immensely since then.

Most often these disease processes, if diagnosed early, are reversible. The person many times returns to normal functioning. That is why a thorough evaluation is so very important when any of these symptoms appear.

Dementia:

A brain disorder caused by the progressive degeneration and death of brain cells.

The following information describing the different types of dementia was taken from information obtained from *Dementia: Not Always Alzheimer's*, published by the Mayo Clinic. I found it very clear and understandable, without becoming too clinically complicated.

Dementia is a neurological disorder that affects a persons ability to think, speak, reason, remember and move. While Alzheimer's disease is the most common dementia, many other conditions can cause these symptoms.

The three most common forms of dementia are Alzheimer's disease, Vascular dementia and Lewey Body dementia. Sometimes the person can have more than one of these problems at the same time.

Vascular Dementia:

Vascular dementia occurs when arteries feeding the brain become narrowed or blocked. The onset of symptoms is abrupt, frequently occurring after a stroke.

Some forms of vascular dementia progress slowly, making them difficult to distinguish from Alzheimer's Disease.

Vascular dementia often causes problems with thinking, language, walking, bladder control and vision. Preventing additional strokes by treating underlying diseases, such as high blood pressure, may halt the progression of vascular dementia.

Lewey Body Dementia:

In this form of dementia, abnormal round structures (Lewey bodies) develop within the cells of the midbrain, beneath the cerebral hemispheres. Lewey Body dementia shares characteristics with both Alzheimer's disease and Parkinson's disease. Like Alzheimer's disease, it causes confusion and impaired memory and judgement. It also produces physical signs typical of Parkinson's disease, shuffling gait and flexed posture. Lewey Body dementia can also cause hallucinations.

Lewey bodies contain a protein associated with Parkinson's disease and Lewey bodies are often found in the brains of people who have Alzheimer's disease. This suggests the three ailments are related, or that Lewey Body dementia and Alzheimer's Disease or Parkinson's Disease sometimes co-exist. Some people with Lewey Body dementia have experienced dramatic improvements in symptoms when treated with Alzheimer's Disease and Parkinson's Disease medications. Several less common brain disorders can also result in dementia.

Frontotemporal Dementia:

Because it affects the lobes of the brain that are responsible for judgement and social behavior, Frontotemporal dementia can result in impolite and socially inappropriate behavior. Symptoms of this form of dementia usually appears between the ages of 40 and 65. The disease seems to run in families.

Pick's Disease:

Pick's Disease is one form of Frontotemporal dementia (FTD). FTD's are a group of rare disorders that affect primarily the frontal and temporal lobes of the brain, which control speech and personality. In Pick's disease, affected areas of the brain contain abnormal brain cells called Pick's bodies. The disease usually occurs in adults between the ages of 40 and 60. The cause is not known.

Unlike Alzheimer's disease in which memory loss usually is the first sign of the problem, people with FTD often show personality changes first. They may become more impulsive and uninhibited, causing them to be socially inappropriate and to make poor decisions. As the disease progresses, they can lose language skills. The disease varies greatly in the way it affects individuals.

There is no cure for Pick's disease. Treatment may include medications and is directed at improving daily function and quality of life. The course of Pick's disease is an inevitable progressive deterioration. The length of progression varies, ranging from less than two years in some to more than 10 years in others. Death is usually caused by infection.

Huntington's Disease:

Symptoms of this hereditary disorder typically begin between the ages of 30 and 50, starting with mild personality changes. As the disorder progresses, a person with Huntington's develops involuntary jerky movements, muscle weakness and clumsiness. Dementia commonly develops in the later stages of the disease.

Parkinson's Disease:

People with Parkinson's disease may experience stiffness of limbs, shaking at rest (tremor), speech impairment and a shuffling gait. Some people with Parkinson's develop dementia late in the disease.

Crutzfeldt-Jacobs Disease:

This extremely rare and fatal brain disorder belongs to a family of human and animal diseases known as the transmissible spongiform encephalopathies. A new variety of Crutzfeldt-Jacobs disease has emerged- particularly in Great Britain. It's believed to be linked to the human consumption of beef from cattle with mad cow disease (bovine spongiform enceopalopathy).

Alzheimer's Disease:

Alzheimer's disease involves a loss of nerve cells in the areas of the brain vital to memory and other mental functions. The loss is associated with the development of abnormal clumps and tangles of protein in brain cells. The first sign of Alzheimer's disease is usually forgetfulness. As the disease progresses, it affects language, reasoning and understanding. Eventually, people with Alzheimer's lose the ability to care for themselves.

The precise cause of Alzheimer's disease is unknown, but risk increases with age. Ten percent of the population over 65 years of age has Alzheimer's disease, while nearly half the population over 85 has the disease.

Alzheimer's disease is the most common form of dementia, affecting about 4.5 million men and women in the United States. Alzheimer's Disease's early symptoms are similar to ones that take place in normal aging. Alzheimer's disease is not a part of normal aging.

TEN WARNING SIGNS

- Recent memory loss affecting job skills
- Difficulty performing familiar tasks
- Problems with language
- Disorientation of time and place
- Poor or decreased judgement
- Problems with abstract thinking
- Misplacing things
- Changes in mood or behavior
- Changes in personality
- Loss of initiative

There is no definitive diagnosis for Alzheimer's disease. The existence of the disease can only be proven at autopsy when the brain tissue can be examined and the plaques and tangles caused by the dead and dying brain cells can be clearly seen.

2

EVALUATION PROCESS
A Diagnosis Of Elimination

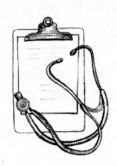

Alzheimer's Disease is a diagnosis of elimination. Meaning that we try to find other reasons for the symptoms in hopes that we find one that may be reversible. Believe me, any one in the medical community when evaluating a potential Alzheimer's disease sufferer prays that they can find something other than the devastating disease of Alzheimer's.

It is very important that the person or family member finds a physician they feel comfortable with. The Neurologist is most likely the usual choice but many family members are more comfortable with their family physicians. Many times the family physician has been seeing this person for years and might be the very one who sees the decline for the first time, Usually as part of their evaluation they will refer you to a Neurologist and maybe even a Psychiatrist.

The Psychiatrist-referral is probably the most alarming to the family and the person suspected of having Alzheimer's disease. Sadly there still remains a stigma about mental illness. Some patients are so afraid that they are going crazy due to the changes in there abilities and memory that they think that others will think the same if they see a Psychiatrist. There is nothing further from the truth. It is usually a combination of physicians that are needed to solve the mystery of these troubling symptoms.

EVALUATION PROCEDURES

Evaluation procedures vary depending on location and available resources. Some are done in a hospital and others done on an out patient basis. Several factors including financial resources have a significant bearing on when, where and to what extent an evaluation is done.

Evaluation components:
Detailed history from someone who knows the person suspected of having Alzheimer's disease and from the person themself to include:

1. Family History of Alzheimer's Disease
2. Education
3. History of Alcohol Consumption
4. Anticholinergic Medications (inhibit acetylcholine action at nerve cell receptors).
5. History of Depression
6. Physical examination
7. Neurological examination
8. Mental status examination
9. Laboratory tests and blood chemistry
10. Thyroid studies
11. VDRL (Venereal Disease Research Laboratories) tests and blood chemistry

12. Lumbar puncture
13. EEG(Electroencephalograph)
14. MRI Scan
15. PET Scan

SELECTING A PHYSICIAN

The primary physician is usually the first doctor that a family will contact when troubling symptoms of memory loss, mood and behavior changes surface.

Since there is no specific doctor for memory, behavior and mood affecting symptoms, the answer rests with a combination of physicians and professionals.

- Geriatrician - One who specializes in Geriatric medicine.

- Neurologist - One who specializes in diseases and conditions of the brain and the nervous system.

- Psychiatrist - One who specializes in conditions that affect mood and behavior.

- Psychologist - One who specializes in the testing of memory and other functions involving mental functions.

Your primary physician can be the one who coordinates the treatment.

Your physician must be patient and understanding. He must be able to spend the time necessary with you and your family to completely understand what symptoms are present and the impact they have on the quality of life of the impaired person and their family. If you do not have this type of relationship with your physician, the Alzheimer's Association may have a list they can share with you of physicians who frequently work with the type of illness.

This relationship with the physician is vitally important to the welfare of your family member. Don't be afraid to ask questions. Bring a list of questions you have, however simple you think they may be. These questions and any added information is invaluable to a physician. They use them to develop a plan of care for your family member. No two patients are alike. Each has individual problems and family dynamics, so please share this information with them. Think of your physicians as detectives. They need all the information and clues you can offer in order to help the Alzheimer's Disease client and their families.

It is understandable that in some cases it may be difficult to obtain a thorough evaluation of a person with Alzheimer's Disease. The family must be able to trust that the doctor they have chosen has done all he can to determine if the disease is present and then rely on his judgement as to the plan of care he suggests.

Studies have shown that an older person is more likely to develop Alzheimer's Disease than a younger person. A person with a family history of the disease is more likely to develop Alzheimer's Disease than a person with no family history of the disease. At this point, no specific risk factors have been identified, however links have been found at a genetic level, such as a gene on chromosome 19 called Apoe-4

The role of Apoe-4 has not been fully understood nor what actually happens to a person if they have this gene. Individuals who have the Apoe-4 gene have developed the disease, and individuals without the gene can also get the disease.

There are two types of Alzheimer's Disease, Familial Alzheimer's Disease (FAD) and sporadic Alzheimer's Disease. The hereditary element is different for each individual. In Familial Alzheimer's Disease, the disease can be traced over several generations. Apparently, familial Alzheimer's Disease is completely inherited. To make it more confusing, apparently there may be a link between genetics and sporadic Alzheimer's Disease.

The research in Alzheimer's Disease continues. I contend there are no real experts in Alzheimer's Disease research or treatment. We are gathering and sharing new information every day. I will always correct anyone who refers to me as an Alzheimer's Disease expert, by virtue of my experience, for this very reason.

I know this is confusing and very frustrating for the Alzheimer's Disease sufferers and their families. They are praying for a cure and so are those of us in the Alzheimer's Disease research, diagnosis and treatment areas.

There are a few protective factors that have been determined:

- Fish or Omega-3 fatty acid
- Mild Alcoholic consumption
- Higher education level
- Regular exercise
- Vitamin C, E, B6 and B12
- Anti - inflammatory therapy
- Statins and Estrogens

Now that we have determined an extensive evaluation is necessary, let's continue presuming that, with our process of elimination, the possibility of Alzheimer's

Disease or a related dementia exists.

The treatment of Alzheimer's Disease is a two fold process. With a better understanding of what the disease is actually doing to the brain and its effect on behavior, both environmental control and selected medications can make it a little easier for the care givers to understand and manage the Alzheimer's Disease and related dementia sufferer. Your physician can suggest the medical interventions as symptoms develop. As we continue you will also learn how, by understanding the disease process and environmental approaches, the caregiver can manage the difficult behavior manifested by the dementia process. It's a team effort.

MEDICATIONS

The National Institute on Aging - Alzheimer's Disease Education & Referral Center lists the latest medication available for the Alzheimer's disease sufferer. The medications are listed in order, as approved by the U.S. Food and Drug Administration, starting with the most recent.

Namenda (Memantine) - prescribed to treat symptoms of moderate to severe Alzheimer's Disease

Razadyne (formerly Reminyl0 (Galantamine)) - prescribed for symptoms of mild to moderate Alzheimer's Disease

Exelon (Rivastigmine) - prescribed to treat symptoms of mild to moderate Alzheimer's Disease

Aricept (Donepezil) - Prescribed to treat symptoms of mild to moderate and moderate to severe Alzheimer's Disease

Cognex (Tacrine) - Prescribed to treat symptoms of

mild to moderate Alzheimer's Disease.

Always consult your prescribing physician to discuss the pros and con of using any of these medications,

As they discuss at the beginning of their article, there are now several medications available to treat symptoms of Alzheimer's disease. They feel, as do I, that treating the symptoms of Alzheimer's disease can provide the disease sufferer with dignity, comfort and independence for a longer period of time, which will be an encouragement for them to continue to assist in their own care, which will be quite a help to their caregivers.

The Alzheimer's Association in your area will always have the latest list of effective medications and research developments.

Remember that the treatment of Alzheimer's Disease uses a combination of approaches.

Understanding behavior management is a primary component of treatment for the Alzheimer's Disease sufferer.

3

ALZHEIMER'S DISEASE PROCESS
It is not your fault

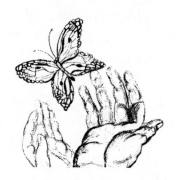

Alzheimer's Disease Facts:

Let us begin our journey of understanding the Alzheimer's Disease process by reviewing the latest facts known about this dreaded disease. We will then proceed to discuss the ramifications of this disease process and the effects they have on the sufferer and the professional and family members who care for them.

Alzheimer's Disease is an irreversible, degenerative brain disease. There is no known cause or cure. Alzheimer's Disease is the number one cause of irreversible dementia. Approximately 4.5 million Americans have Alzheimer's Disease. Alzheimer's Disease strikes in all socioeconomic classes and ethnic groups. Alzheimer's Disease effects women more than men. This may be due to women living longer than men.

Alzheimer's Disease is not normal aging. However, the risk of developing the disease increases with each decade of life - 20 % of 65 year olds, 50 % of those 85 and older. Alzheimer's Disease is the fourth lead-ing cause of death, behind heart disease, cancer and stroke.

There is progressive deterioration over time from 2 to 20 years. Death usually is a result of pneumonia or overwhelming infection. Approximately 20 % of nursing home residents have Alzheimer's Disease. Cost for care exceeds twenty billion dollars per year (Alzheimer's Association of Sarasota and Manatee Counties).

As mentioned in Alzheimer's Disease Facts, it is a degenerative disease of the brain. It destroys the cells of the brain, and with them, its ability to function in order to retain memories, abilities and intellect. It initially affects the frontal lobe, temporal lobe and the speech centers. Ultimately, it will effect the entire brain.

The neurons are needed for transferring messages from one area of the brain to the other. The neurons communicate with each other by crossing a gap called a synapse. Its much like the current traveling along an electrical cord. In order for the impulse to travel to the next neuron, it must pick up the neurotransmitters needed to continue its journey across the synapse.

The disease process is destroying the neurotransmitter necessary to allow the impulse to travel. This neurotransmitter is called Acetylcholine. Let's liken it to Sarasota Bay. There are boats on one side of the bay waiting to get across, but there is no water in the bay. There is no way for the boats to get to the other side. Therefore the messages are not getting through. Eventually destroying the brains capacity for storing any new information. We hear information process it and store it for retrieval later. This process of storing information is called encoding.

This inability to encode new information is why so many care givers complain of having to repeat information over and over again to their loved one with Alzheimer's disease. If the message is finally understood, the disease sufferer cannot store this information so later that day the care giver finds themselves having to repeat the process again. The Alzheimer's disease sufferer may also repeat statements over and over again because they cannot remember saying them.

Let's liken it to a computer. The monitor and the key board are there. The message is heard and typed on the keyboard, but when the enter key is pressed the message cannot be processed. When the save process is selected, the computer can no longer complete this request.

Along with destroying the brains ability to store any new information, it is also destroying all the remaining information stored in the brain, memories, abilities and any knowledge acquired throughout the person's lifetime.

Imagine if you will that the wall across the room you are sitting in contains all that you are as a human being. Alzheimer's Disease systematically erases all of that information from your brain.

In the early stages, it removes scattered patches of intellect, memory, judgment and daily routines. As it continues, it erases language, self care abilities and bodily functions, as it destroys the brain.

As the disease progresses, the person regresses. They are going backwards in time. The person loses all abilities until the only functions that are left are those of a new born child curled up in a fetal position. The Alzheimer's Disease sufferer is left without the abilities to survive. Unable to eat, speak or perform normal function, to the extent that the body forgets how to nourish itself. Foods given are passed through the body without the ability to send the nutrients to the needed areas.

Let me use myself as an example. What if I had Alzheimer's Disease? God Forbid! I am always compelled to say that whenever I begin this example. Alzheimer's Disease is such a devastating disease. I am a sixty one year old woman, married for forty years to a handsome 6' 2" Irishman with sparkling blue eyes and freckles, named Jim. I have a thirty six year old son, Mike, who strongly resembles me. Mike is married to a lovely girl named Susan.

Mike's resemblance to me is so strong that whenever I tried to sneak on to the school yard, when I had yard duty, I was always discovered, much to my embarrassment. Let me explain.

Mike was a very active, adventuresome child. Always a challenge for a Catholic school's structured environment. Invariably, I would come onto the schoolyard to discover that one of the sisters already had my son in tow. Scolding him for yet another indiscretion. I can't imagine where he got that from! As I came onto the school yard, one of the other sisters would come up to me and say, "You're Michael's mom aren't you?" - in a most accusatory tone, I might add. I felt the urge to apologize for my over- zealous son, but I didn't. I loved his zest for life and still do.

I was born and raised in Pennsylvania. My parents were Italian. I lived in a three-story, double-brick home. I have two sisters. My father and mother are both dead now. I am called Sandy most often by friends and Sandra by my family. My maiden name was DeMatteo. A far cry from Kehoe isn't it?

Alzheimer's Disease has caused me to regress to the point that I think I am 20 years old. Sure would like to have that firm body again, but I digress. I might also pass a mirror and begin to talk to that person I see in the mirror. Another sad but interesting aspect of this regression process. The person's face I see in the mirror is my mother's. I expected to see my 20 year old face. We will talk about that in greater depth in the chapter on behavior management.

At 20 years old, I lived at home, my parents were still alive, I wasn't married and I didn't have any children.

The problem is that now I live in Sarasota, Florida. If I walked outside and turned away from the door I just exited, I would not be able to find my way back. I would begin to walk down the street, looking for the home I remember. A very frightening experience for me and my family.

Do to these all to frequent escapades and the fact that I refused to let strangers care for me, including my husband, my family has found it necessary to place me in a specialized, safe environment. A staff member approaches me and says, "Mrs. Kehoe, your husband is here to see you." I appreciate the young lady speaking to me but who is Mrs. Kehoe? Such a sweet girl. She always smiles at me and talks to me in such a kind, soft voice.

In front of me, now, is a very attractive older man. I know I know him; I can feel it. But how? He's calling me Sandy. He surely knows me. He can't be my husband. I'm not married. He's too old for me anyway! He isn't Italian, that's for sure. He must be my uncle. There's a young man with him. He says, "Hi Mom! Its me, Mike." That's strange. How could I be his mom.

I'm too young. I feel so strongly about him. Boy, he really looks a lot like me. I have two sisters. He must be my cousin. I am so glad they are visiting me. I must be important to them.

What a traumatic experience for my husband of forty years. "Why would my wife not remember me? Was I not a good husband? Did she ever really love me?" Then there's my son who thinks I have erased him from my memory completely. "How could my mom just forget me?"

The only comfort they would have is knowing that it is the disease process and not them that is at fault A subject often discussed in family support groups. Hopefully they have been attending the support group offered by the Alzheimer's Association of Manatee and Sarasota counties. A support group may be meeting in the same facility that I live in. How lucky for my family.

They will realize that I know and love the people in my life. But their presence in my life will have to be according to where I am at the moment. They will have to enter my world. I may not know exactly who they are to me now, but I do know I love them, and they are important to me and should continue visiting me.

This is one of the most important lessons a family member can learn. So many times the family members feel that it is something that they did wrong that makes the Alzheimer's Disease sufferer treat them as if they don't know them. It was experiencing one of these occasions that has given me the impetus to continue educating the community.

While explaining the regression associated with this disease I noticed a young women in the audience crying. After completing the lecture, I walked up to her and asked her why she was crying. She explained to me that her mother had Alzheimer's Disease. Her mother didn't recognize her any more. She believed that she must have been a terrible child not to have left a memory of her with her mother. She now realized that it was not her fault and that she can relate to her mother again by simply entering her world. I knew then that I must never stop educating the community, until every spouse, child and family is relieved of this sadness.

The following information was received from the Alzheimer's Association. I think it really helps care givers understand the situation they find themselves in. It simply encourages them to:

Remember

You are entering the world of now!

There is no yesterday

There is no tomorrow

There is only now

STAGES

There are several opinions as to the stages of the Alzheimer's disease process. Some choose to discuss the disease in a 7 stages process.

Others, like myself, look at it in a simpler context. Three stages: Beginning or Early Stage, Middle Stage and Late or Final Stage. It is also very important to remember that each Alzheimer's disease sufferer is an individual. Stages may overlap.

I cared for a lovely southern lady who was relatively clear early in the day. As the day progressed she became more confused and mentally younger in age. Towards the evening hours she became very agitated and tearful.

She suffered with sun downers syndrome. We will discuss this in greater detail in the chapter covering behavior management. As the person goes through the day and becomes tired and maybe overstimulated by the days activities, they become more confused.

When helping her dress for the day, she would ask where her mother was. We would tell her that her mother was in heaven. Being a very religious person, she would be satisfied with this answer. As the day progressed and she became more confused, the same question would be asked. At that time, we would tell her that her mother was fine and would see her tomorrow. You see, in the early to late afternoon this sweet gentile women became a child. We could not use the same answer that we used in the morning.

The symptoms seem to progress in a pattern and this order of stages provides a way to understand the progression of the disease.

1. Beginning or Early Stage:

The early stage is a stage that the person may be able to perceive. They know that something is wrong. They are becoming forgetful. The ability to store recent memories is lost.

Their daily routines become difficult to manage. It begins to affect language especially nouns. They forget names. Forget to pay bills. The homes may be very messy, filled with debris and unopened mail. There refrigerators may have little food in them, as they frequently forget to shop.

They begin to forget how to operate the appliances in their kitchens. They may have a can and a can opener and cannot remember how they are used together. This is called apraxia. To be able to recognize these items, the information about them has to be recalled from stored memory. An ability the disease sufferer is rapidly losing.

They begin to forget procedures at work or even the familiar route to their job. Losing things becomes a problem, because they forget that they have lost them. That's the difference with the stress induced forgetfulness. We know that we have misplaced our glasses, for an example, and we will eventually remember where we put the them.

A young woman came up to me after the session about the early stage of Alzheimer's Disease. She told me that her mother lived out of State and when she called her she sounded fine and told her all about the meeting she went to at church. She knew she was becoming a little forgetful, but she felt she was still safe. Just to make sure, she set up meals on wheels to ensure that her mom was eating well.

When the meals were brought to her mothers home, she smiled at the delivery person and said that her daughter was such a worrier, "She was Fine." Luckily the person from Meals on Wheels looked around and saw how messy the woman's home was. She asked if she could leave the meal anyway, since she had no one else to bring it to. The woman agreed. As the woman opened the refrigerator, she noticed there wasn't anything in it except spoiled milk.

The group handling the Meals on Wheels contacted the daughter and told her what they had found. When the daughter phoned some of her mom's friends, they said that they hadn't seen her mom recently, since she had stopped attending church meetings.

Many times the families don't realize the extent of the deficits until something like this happens. It can be two years into the process of the disease before a family member discovers the problem. This is not uncommon.

The Alzheimer's Disease sufferer may even become reclusive, not wanting their family and friends to find out. If they were attending church meetings regularly or was an avid card player, suddenly they stop attending. They forget to pay bills. They may be tricked into buying things they don't need or even swindled out of a life fortune by unscrupulous people, due to their poor judgment. They may be still driving but due to a poor spacial awareness get lost easily or may even be driving on the wrong side of the street.

This is the most dangerous stage for the person and the most problematic for the family, as they become aware. It is difficult to intervene, since the person becomes very adept at bridging to cover up their symptoms and will vehemently deny any problems. Many families have had to disable the family car or remove it altogether to prevent the person from driving. Many have had to take over the finances to protect their parents financially.

Denial of the existence of a problem makes it difficult for family members to help. The affected persons are very paranoid and do not want anyone handling their affairs. They may have frequent mood swings and anger easily as the ability to bridge the deficits becomes harder for them This stage can go on for two to four years from the onset of symptoms.

As I was relating these symptoms to a group of police officers who were attending a workshop offered by the local Alzheimer's Association, one of the detectives looked suddenly saddened. I asked him later what had affected him so, and he related this story to me.

He explained that he had just assisted in an eviction of an elderly woman. Now because of the description I gave of an early Alzheimer's sufferer, he feels that the woman was probably suffering from Alzheimer's Disease. He further explained that they were sent because she had not been paying her bills or her taxes. Her house was filled with debris and unopened mail. As they were trying to clear things out of her house, she was bringing it back in a little cart. He remembers his young colleague scolding the elderly women for doing so but it didn't stop her. The officer explained that he was now concerned for her welfare, and after the session, he would make sure he found out what happened to her and make sure she was somewhere safe.

2. Middle Stage:

In the middle stage, there is increasing memory loss, confusion and shortened attention span. It is harder for them to recognize close friends or family. They become more restless especially in the late afternoon or evening. (sun downing).

The person may become irritable, fidgety or the emotions become more labile, crying or laughing unexpectedly.

Their personal care becomes sloppy. They may be wearing the wrong thing for the season or several outfits at the same time. They can also forget the order that clothing belongs. A gentleman might put his underwear on over his trousers.

They forget the sequence of actions to complete the task. This is called agnosia. They may find the bathroom but can't remember if they sit down first or take they pants down. Their care giver may ask them to sit down, but they cannot get their bodies to respond. Remember? The message cannot move along the nerve tract. They may know what they want to do, but their bodies will not respond, because their brain cannot send the message.

Showing the person exactly what is expected of them is very helpful at this stage. If you want them to sit down, pat the chair or sit down yourself. Remember though, a gentleman from the old school does not sit down until the lady does. If a woman gets up, he may get up as well, out of respect. This disease, though very sad, is fascinating. One discovers how much our past can help someone understand why we react as we do in situations that come up in this disease process.

In one of the facilities that I served as a Alzheimer's Unit Director, we were having a dance for our residents. One man who was having great difficulty walking at this stage suddenly came up to me, took me onto the dance floor and led me around the floor, expertly doing the steps appropriate for the music being played. Seeing the other people dancing added a great visual cue for him as well. We were all amazed. The staff surrounded us, as he moved with the grace of Fred Astaire. I was just trying to keep step with him. He had selected the only person in the room with two left feet for his partner, I'm afraid. They clapped as he performed. He was so proud. He was somebody again. Tears ran down our faces.

When the music stopped, he couldn't even get off the dance floor safely. I had to support him, as we left the dance floor. I don't think he minded though, all he could hear and experience was the applause he received, as he left the dance floor.

We found out that he was a dance instructor as a young man and loved to dance every chance he got. His wife had not mentioned it, since it was so long ago. A thorough history of likes and dislikes, talents and skills should be taken when caring for an Alzheimer's disease sufferer. Those areas of the brain may be able to respond to the right stimuli. This information is invaluable when the care givers are trying to help the disease sufferer comprehend a message, and it also allows the care giver to better understand the person's reaction to certain circumstances.

The music brought back the skills and balance that he had lost. That area of his brain could function with the right stimuli. It always made me think of Mel Tellis. He has great difficulty speaking, since he has had a severe stuttering problem since childhood, except when he was singing.

The person begins to sleep more often. If a person sleeps too much during the day, he may have a tendency to get up and wander at night. It is important to try and keep the person occupied during the day, so they will be tired at night.

I can hear you saying, "That's easy for you to say." but, believe me, with some of the approaches we will discuss later, this can be accomplished. We will discuss some beneficial activities in future chapters.

They may hear or see things that are not there. Especially in the Lewy - Body type of dementia. This can be very frightening for the family or spouse. This reaction, as discussed before, can be a medication reaction or a sign that the person is ill. Make sure you inform the physician of any sudden changes. If none of those problems exist, try to go along with the person, as long as the hallucination is not a frightening or dangerous one.

Many care givers find it difficult to agree with the person who is hallucinating. Some mental health professionals even think this is reinforcing a delusion, but in this case, it is not. If you are uncomfortable with agreeing that you see whatever they are seeing, you may answer the person by saying, "I believe you see that; I just cannot see it." It can be much more frightening for the disease sufferer if you disagree. Remember! The person really sees whatever they are telling you they see.

I once cared for a client who believed little children lived in her room with her. We had to be careful where we sat in her room when we came in to visit her. Invariably, one of us would attempt to sit in one of the chairs in her room and, wouldn't you know it, that chair was the very one the children were sitting on. We would apologize and find another seat. We will be discussing other interventions later.

The brain of the Alzheimer's sufferer can also alter what they are seeing. The loss of brain function has altered their perception of the world around them. It can become difficult for them to maneuver themselves to a chair and sit down. This loss of perception can also interfere with their ability to read and write their names.

The person may also try to undress or relieve themselves in inappropriate places. They cannot find the bathroom anymore. A scheduled toileting program may solve both of these problems. We will discuss other interventions in the next few chapters.

The person may begin hiding their possessions or accusing their spouses of infidelity, as they are becoming very suspicious and paranoid.

They have increased appetites. And may want increased amounts of food, since they cannot remember when or if they have eaten. Junk foods may become their favorites. If the disease sufferer is in a facility at this point, they may even tell their families that they haven't had a thing to eat all day. When you check with their care givers, the families invariably find out their family member had all of their meals and probably several snacks that day.

In a facility I managed, we had a very skillful young lady who would stand by the food delivery cart and eat all the desserts if we didn't catch her in time.

If the disease sufferer does not have diabetes or any other disorder that would prohibit this increased consumption of food, don't worry about it. The extra pounds they may put on will serve them well when they reach the final stages, where the body can no longer store nutrients from food.

Remember, even with these diminished abilities, people with Alzheimer's disease, at this stage, think they are alright and behaving normally. Mercifully, at this stage, they do not realize the abilities they have lost. They believe they are still somebody. They are not doing these things on purpose!

I have learned many wonderful things from the many Alzheimer's Disease sufferers I have taken care of. The most important is not to underestimate the worth of any person. Even with diminished abilities, a person has great worth.

And so it was with our "Butterfly." She was a diminutive, five-foot tall, little lady, weighing a total of ninety pounds. Dementia had stripped her of many of her abilities, even her ability to communicate, but she could still walk around safely. She could, however, say one sentence, "I love you." She would walk among her fellow residents and care staff, touch them lightly on their arm or hand and say, "I love you."

When she would notice her family members coming in the door, she would raise her arm and wave at them saying, "I love you." This simple act was such a wonderful gift for her family and my staff.

Suddenly, one day, she collapsed to the floor. Apparently, in addition to the dementia, she had a severe heart condition. Her heart had simply ceased to function. Our *Butterfly* was gone.

At her memorial, her family mentioned that her habit of calling out, "I love you," to them, as they arrived and left her presence, was a life long habit. Apparently, Alzheimer's Disease had taken away almost everything except her gift of love.

I find myself telling my family how much I love them every day. This little person had changed many of our lives forever.

This stage is the longest one and may last two to ten years after diagnosis.

3. End or Final Stage:

The ability to recognize family members and even themselves in the mirror is impaired by this stage. As they regress in time, the persons they see may be much younger in their memory now. As I had explained earlier, when I used myself as an example, I would be expecting to see my twenty year old face, not my mothers. Remember they know you belong to them and still love you. They must try and place you in the time and place they are now.

The weight loss will begin to become apparent now. Even with more frequent meals. Difficulty swallowing may appear at this point as well. Total assistance with their meals becomes necessary. They may become emaciated. The brain deterioration has destroyed their bodies ability to process food and use the nutrients efficiently.

The person has lost the ability for self care and may also lose the ability to control their bladder and bowels. If the disease sufferer is not in a care facility at this point, the incontinence is usually the symptoms that convinces the family that professional care may be needed.

The ability to communicate orally at this point may be completely lost. Watch their facial expressions for clues of their condition. Please, please, continue to visit and discuss your activities and the family news with your family member. Touch them on the hand. They'll know you are there and that you love them, even if they can no longer respond to you. Hearing and the sense of touch are the last senses to leave a person, as they are dying.

In an Alzheimer's facility I managed in Sarasota, one of our residents was in the very last stage of her disease process. She was drifting away quickly. The family wanted her to have a priest visit her in her last hours. At this point, she was no longer responding to her family or staff. We didn't even suspect she knew we were there with her. We were so wrong!

When the priest came to visit her and began to recite the Our Father, she began to say it with him. He was visibly shaken, as he did not expect any response from her.

As she recited the *Our Father*, though her eyes were closed, tears streamed down her face. She died shortly after the priest's visit, with her family at her bedside.

There will be more frequent infections, and they may experience seizures. The disease sufferer will also sleep more and may become comatose.

The Alzheimer's disease sufferer usually dies with Alzheimer's Disease, not from the disease. It is usually pneumonia or an over all sepsis(Infection) that causes their death.

As described earlier, if the person actually survives to this stage of the disease process, their functions would be those of a newborn child curled up in a fetal position and left without the ability to survive. That information has been destroyed. They may become comatose and eventually die.

4

COMMUNICATION
"Listen to me, I am still Somebody"

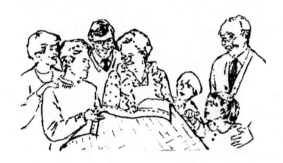

Alzheimer's disease destroys the sufferers ability to communicate. At first it causes the memory loss of nouns or name words. The person may want a specific item but cannot remember its name. This can be very frustrating and embarrassing for the disease sufferer.

The disease process continues to destroy the ability to form comprehensive sentences. At this time, in order to understand, you must observe the persons gestures, facial expressions and their body language to determine what they are trying to say. Not to be humorous, but it becomes much like playing charades. If you are good at that, you will have no trouble understanding the Alzheimer's disease sufferer at this stage. Finally, speech may become garbled or completely absent.

The most important lesson one has to learn, at this point, is that the disease sufferer is desperately trying to communicate with you. They want to be heard. It helps them to feel as if they have worth. Actually, the sub title of this chapter and the title of this book was taken from an article I wrote for the Alzheimer's

Association in Houston, Texas many years ago. It was written, describing an actual event in my life, in an attempt to explain the need for the Alzheimer's disease sufferer to communicate and be listened to.

"LISTEN TO ME, I AM STILL SOMEBODY"
Communicating with the Alzheimer's Disease Patient

A SIMPLE CONCEPT

Since I have been in the field of Alzheimer's Disease patient care, my understanding of basic communication has changed dramatically.

I have come to the conclusion that it is not the content of the message that is the most important factor. It is the fact that someone is listening to you that gives what you say importance and you a feeling of self worth.

As a young mother, I was taught this very concept by my then three-year-old son, Mike. Mike and I would visit my grandmother every Saturday afternoon. Mike loved his great-grandmother. He called her Grammy.

One may suspect the visit might have been self-serving on Mike's part. All great-grandmothers have special treats on hand should their great-grandchildren visit. Grammy was no exception. She had a crystal bowl filled with candy, Twinkies and 7-UP in the kitchen. Twinkies and 7-UP were Grammy's favorites as well.

During these visits, Mike would sit on the floor beside Grammy's chair, and they would watch wrestling together. Grammy loved wrestling, next to Lawrence Welk of course. By the way, Mike knew that cartoons came on right after wrestling.

It was so entertaining watching the two of them. Grammy would leap from her chair to chastise her favorite wrestler and Mike would be right beside her following her every move.

During this visit, their conversation was particularly lively and animated. Grammy would lean over the side of her chair and say something to Mike, and then they would throw back their heads, laughing heartily.

My grandmother was born in Italy. She came to this country when she was eighteen to marry my grandfather. She spoke only "broken English." She would expertly capture your attention with a few English words and quickly revert to her native language. Speaking Italian was much easier for her now, as she approached her ninety third year.

How wonderful, I thought. My son was learning Italian. I always regretted not learning Italian myself.

When the wrestling match was over, Grammy went to her room for her afternoon nap. I called Mike over and told him how pleased I was that he was learning Italian. He gave me a very puzzled look. "Mommy, what was Grammy saying?" That question was my first realization that Mike, although appearing to converse with his great-grandmother, had not understood a word she said.

"I thought you understood Grammy." "No, Mommy, when she shook her head, I shook my head, when she frowned, I frowned." Actually, Mike didn't use the word frown. He said, "When her face did this. I did it too." I can still see his sweet little face all wrinkled up to demonstrate. "When she smiled, I smiled." He concluded.

How Simple! How very Simple!

Children are so wonderfully perceptive and non judgmental. They are able to see things so clearly. They accept without hesitation. We adults would be doing well to follow their example.

I did not realize how significant this touching scenario would become for me in the years to come.

It wasn't surprising that Mike was one of Grammy's favorite great grandchildren. Not because he could understand Italian, but because with a child's innocence, he made her feel like someone special. He gave her his time and loving attention. He listened! You see, it is not only the Alzheimer's Disease sufferers who have this need. We all do.

Alzheimer's Disease robs its sufferers of their basic language skills, especially in the later stages. They are trying to communicate, even though their conversation is fragmented and confusing. It may make no sense to us, but it does to them. They feel their message is very clear and deserves to be listened to. We simply have to listen actively, watching their expressions and body language for clues. We all need to feel special. Listening to our Alzheimer's Disease patients makes them feel as if they are important and what they say has worth.

What a simple gift.

I have had the pleasure of speaking to many groups of care givers, both family and professional. I have used this very true story many times. I thank my now thirty four-year-old son and the many Alzheimer's Disease sufferers for my understanding of communication.

"The eyes of men converse as much as their tongues, with the advantage that the ocular dialect needs no dictionary but is understood the world over," Ralph Waldo Emerson.

Thanks to my son, a lesson I learned years ago.

While we are awaiting the answers research may bring, let us use the simple things: Respect for our patients, understanding of their special needs and a loving acceptance of them as important individuals, with something worthwhile to say.

"It's ok if you can no longer remember the words or how to use them correctly. What you have to say is important to me. I'm listening! I love you." This particular part of my book is very important. Without understanding communication, one cannot begin to manage the difficult behavior we will be discussing in the next chapter.

I will simplify the concept by discussing each aspect of the process individually:

VERBAL

Begin the conversation by identifying yourself and calling the person by name.

This action relieves the anxiety caused by not knowing your name. We have all experienced this one. All of a sudden someone comes up to you and starts talking to you, and you have no idea who they are. You are so afraid they will find out you can't remember their name that you don't have a clue what they are talking about. The same thing happens to the Alzheimer's disease sufferer. They do not want to be embarrassed either.

Calling the person by name assures them you are someone they must know. As I have mentioned before, using their last name, although polite, may not be beneficial. The best approach is to use their first name.

In my case, if you called me Sandra Marie I would think that I was in trouble. My mother would use my entire name,when she was about to scold me. Sandy is a more disarming way to address me.

That can be a nickname - like Coach, when a man was a highschool or college coach. The family can be a great source of information at this time.

We had a very difficult patient to manage. We tried everything. Not until the family told us he was in the military did we have any success. Apparently, he was a Captain in the Marines. We began to call him Captain or Sir. We discussed the activities as if we were in the military too. "Sir, It's time for supper. Lets go to the chow hall," "Let's go to the parade grounds for a walk," and so forth. We will discuss these interventions further in the chapter on dealing with difficult behaviors.

Use specific and familiar words:

This does not mean baby talk. That would be offensive and insulting to the person. Remember, they think they are thinking clearly. As with the military person we discussed earlier, we used military terms he was familiar with. They cannot think in the abstract, so do not joke; they won't get it. Do explain all procedures as simply as possible, before you attempt them.

Use short, simple sentences:

"Come here," preferably while gesturing with your hand. "Sit here," while pointing to the chair or patting the seat. "Its time to eat now," as opposed to,"Come into the dining room. Its time for dinner, and I don't want it to get cold." (Way too many words! The

Alzheimer's disease sufferer lost you at, "...come into the dining room.")

NONVERBAL

Stand face to face:

The person does not know you are speaking to them, unless you are looking directly at them, and it also helps them to comprehend your message.

A frustrated care giver once told me she just thought her husband was ignoring her. " He never listened to me anyway." She was obviously very offended by this behavior. She was relieved to hear that it wasn't his intent. She just had not gotten his complete attention.

Maintain eye contact:

If the Alzheimer's Disease sufferer is seated, make sure you stoop down or sit beside then before you begin your conversation. Standing over someone when you are conversing with them can be very intimidating. It can make the person very anxious. Eye contact also makes the job of comprehending your message much easier for the disease sufferer.

Move slowly:

Sudden movements can startle the person. They may perceive it as a hostile action and strike at you.

Sadly, this simple action can label an Alzheimer's disease sufferer as combative. This label is not deserved, in many situations. Usually, it happens because of our actions while trying to communicate. This can lead to the use of medications to reduce aggressive behavior, before they are actually necessary. When all other interventions have failed, the use of these medications can be very useful in helping both

the professional and family care giver manage the behaviors. Let's not label a person too soon.

Touch the person on the hand or arm:

A touch on the hand or arm can be very reassuring
and emphasize the message.

I am Italian and find myself compelled to touch everyone on the hand or arm, when I am talking to them.
I am also a hugger, so beware. This approach would
be very easy for me, however it is not appreciated by
everyone. In some nationalities, it is actually offensive.
The person takes it as an act of disrespect. I really try
hard to control this impulse.

The Alzheimer's disease sufferer may have these
same feelings or fear close contact. When attempting to communicate, begin to take a step forward. If
the person steps back, its an indication they are uncomfortable and probably would not appreciate being touched. They are guarding their personal space.
Watch their behavior closely.

Use facial expressions and gestures for emphasis:

Yet another intervention I seem to have no problem with. We Italians frequently gesture when we are
talking. Actually, if my hands were held, I probably
wouldn't be able to speak at all.

It is not as easy for everyone. People are not used
to making faces and gesturing wildly just to have their
message understood. Knowing this, when I addressed
a class of fledgling therapists, after explaining this approach, I took the class into a room where a therapist
was attempting to encourage a group of Alzheimer's
Disease clients to exercise - a difficult task at best for
any exercise instructor. The class noticed that if the

therapist wanted the clients to exercise, she had to do the exercise as well. Jumping jacks, marching in place and touching their toes were all being demonstrated by the therapist. The students were to assist in this endeavor. They were to put into use the interventions they had just learned. The encounter was very enlightening. They also noticed that the therapist was in great shape.

STYLE

Speak slowly:

Rapid fire speech patterns make the message very hard to comprehend. Slow down your speech pattern and enunciate each word. It's a gift your disease sufferer will appreciate.

Speak softly:

Loud talking, when talking to the Alzheimer's sufferer, can be startling and cause unnecessary anxiety. It denotes anger and makes the person uneasy. They feel they are being scolded for some wrong doing. Remember, they are regressing in age; it's a natural reaction for the child they have become.

Ask one question at a time:

If you ask to many questions at a time, you stop the processing of the original question. Each new question stops the previous process and begins it anew, in an attempt to process the new message. It delays the comprehension of the messages and is frustrating for the Alzheimer's disease sufferer and the sender of the message.

If you have to repeat a message, repeat it exactly:

This concept is particularly difficult for educators. They are taught that if the student cannot comprehend the subject matter, repeat it in a different context. This is not the approach that works for the disease sufferer.

When anyone begins to talk to the Alzheimer's Disease sufferer, it initiates the message processing. It takes about ten seconds for a response. The processing takes a little while to accomplish. If after ten seconds there is no response, repeat your message, exactly. If the words are changed, the original message is dropped and the new message begins to be processed. Don't rush them. This approach is a good test of patience for the care givers but an invaluable one when trying to get the disease sufferer to comply with your wishes. Armed with this information we can proceed to the chapters concerning behavior management and behavior management techniques.

5

BEHAVIOR MANAGEMENT
Every action causes a reaction

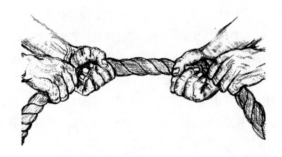

The order of my chapters is very telling. It displays my particular understanding of the techniques necessary to care for the Alzheimer's Disease sufferer.

I contend that one cannot have an effect on the disease sufferer's behavior without understanding the disease process itself. Nor can the caregiver manage behavior without thoroughly understanding the communication techniques necessary to help the disease sufferer comprehend and process the messages their care givers are sending.

Much of the behaviors exhibited by the Alzheimer's Disease sufferer is linked to their reaction to their environment. Remember science class? Here's a gem that I never thought I would resurrect again. Every action has an equal or opposite reaction. This fact explains much of the behaviors of the Alzheimer's sufferer. They are reacting to their environment and our actions. They do not initiate behavior just to be troublesome. Sadly, the process this would take is no longer functioning. They may have an accident and urinate in an inappropriate place. Not because they are lazy, but because they can no longer find the bathroom or follow the sequence of actions necessary to relieve themselves properly.

We were at a workshop and a care giver raised her hand to complain that her mother, who was living with her since she could no longer live alone safely, was creating "a nuisance of herself and a bad example for her grand children." Apparently she would go into the bathroom (At least she could still find it), make a mess of the toilet paper, when wiping herself, and usually come out of the bathroom trailing toilet paper behind her. Sound like any child you might know? Remember, the person is regressing.

Anyway, the daughter said she was so frustrated with her mother's behavior and asked if we could share anything with her, so she could stop her mother from doing these annoying things.

The answer to her question was not what she expected. One could see it from her reaction. She was told that her mother couldn't control this behavior. She should toilet her mother on a routine basis to avoid the necessity of her mother trying to care for herself. The responsibility of changing behavior rests with the care giver.

The Alzheimer's Disease sufferer can no longer correctly locate themselves in time and space and cannot recognize simple objects or operate equipment safely.

This includes driving a car. Though driving skills may remain, the sense of where you are on the road becomes impaired. Going the wrong way on a one way street, for example. The ability to perceive a dangerous situation is greatly impaired as are their reaction times in these situations.

A gentleman in the early to middle stages of the disease process insisted on driving, although his wife realized he was no longer safe. She tried to convince him to let her drive, but he refused. He was a large and imposing man, and she was afraid to push him further. Finally, she was too afraid to travel with him. Luckily!

One day, he left the house, got lost and drove onto a bridge under construction. There were large girders on flat bed trucks parked at the entrance of the construction site. Not seeing them, he drove into the back of one of these flatbed trucks. A steel girder came through his front windshield over the passenger side of the car and continued to the back seat. The very seat his wife would have been occupying, if she had accompanied him that day.

He was uninjured and unaware of the actions that had caused this accident. Due to this accident, his physician wrote a letter to the bureau of motor vehicles and requested that his license be revoked. This procedure is often used by care givers, because it takes the onus off of them, and the disease sufferer seems to be able to accept it easier from an official person.

Interestingly enough, in the earlier stages, the truth works the best or at least a statement that makes sense to them is more easily accepted. Do not lie. If you need an excuse for the car not being there, say that a family member had to use it. That makes sense. One family member told the disease sufferer that his car had been stolen. He simply called his dealership and ordered a new one. Boy! Was that salesman disappointed when the family had to cancel the sale.

Remember, the Alzheimer's Disease sufferer does not realize the destruction of the disease or its affect on their thinking processes. Their judgment is severely impaired even though, in the earlier stages, their physical abilities may not be.

Illness can affect the behavior as well. As I had mentioned earlier, the symptoms of illness or distress may not be apparent to the care giver. The disease sufferer may have pain but cannot express it. By the way, the Alzheimer's disease sufferer does feel pain. So many times I hear both professional care givers and family care givers say a person with Alzheimer's Disease cannot feel pain. There is nothing further from the truth.

This is an interesting problem though, since a care giver may not realize that the change in behavior may be due to pain or illness. In trying to teach a group of care givers how they might be able to recognize these sometimes subtle changes, I would use this as an simple gauge.

If the person with Alzheimer's Disease is usually a happy person and their behavior is manageable and suddenly they become agitated and difficult to manage, they are probably ill. Conversely, if an Alzheimer's disease sufferer is usually a challenge and suddenly becomes compliant, he is probably ill, as well, even though this calm behavior may be a relief to the care giver. Seemingly unexplained fears can cause difficult, uncontrollable behavior as well. Many times we have to investigate the person's past in order to find the answers to unusual unprovoked behavior.

One such occasion, was described in an Alzheimer's Disease presentation I attended during a conference in Florida. Every afternoon, about three o'clock in the afternoon, one of the residents in a facility began screaming. There was no way she could be comforted. The facility tried to figure out what the problem was.

They watched what was happening each day at that time. Apparently, there was a male nurse who came onto the unit at that same time every day. They assumed she was afraid of him. He was almost investigated for abuse, but the family of the resident stepped in. The family said they had noticed he was wearing hard soled shoes and had a very heavy step. The family informed the facility Administration that their mother was a Holocaust survivor. The heavy step probably reminded her of the German soldiers who had imprisoned her and brought back the terror of those years. The male nurse changed to soft soled shoes. The behavior vanished with the shoes.

Now, I don't mean to suggest that every behavior will be as easily resolved but it is surprising how, with a little investigation, we can resolve some very difficult behavior.

Remember the Alzheimer's Disease sufferer does not initiate behavior. They are reacting to their environment or some other stimulus.

When I was in Houston, working for the Alzheimer's Assoc., I received a call from a frantic care giver. He explained that his wife was saying there were men outside in the front yard trying to take out their tree. I asked the husband if anything had happened in the past that concerned the tree. He explained to me that about ten years ago he had a tree planted in the front yard as a surprise for his wife. I explained to him that this may be what she is seeing. Just tell her that it was a surprise for her.

Many family members find it difficult to go along with an Alzheimer's disease sufferer, when they are hallucinating. That's ok. You can just say, "I believe you see that, I just cannot see it myself."

Do not argue. They are really seeing it. The brain stores everything we have experienced, seen or learned, much like a video recorder. As the disease continues to destroy the brain and its contents, it replays some of these experiences or memories. The person may see their young children running around the house.

The hallucinations can also come from something the person has recently seen on television. As the disease progresses, the ability to distinguish real life from television becomes very difficult.

If a story about a robbery or a fire has just been televised, the person may believe it is happening to him.

If, however the person sees something that frightens him, he may try to protect himself, putting the care giver in harms way. Many times, watching TV can be the frightening stimuli.

Watching TV would appear to be an activity that could not possibly bother the Alzheimer's Disease sufferer; but it most definitely is. The Alzheimer's Disease sufferer cannot differentiate between television and real life, especially in the middle stages. They believe the person on the TV is in the room with them. We have had clients actually punch at the screen in an attempt to stop the person on TV from talking.

Many times what the disease sufferer sees on TV will be replayed later, especially if it was a frightening newscast. Of course, to the dismay of the care giver, it is usually in the middle of the night, when they awake frightened, that what they saw is happening to them, causing many sleepless nights for them and their care givers. This is why it is important for the care giver and many persons hired to care for the Alzheimer's Disease sufferer to have had training about Alzheimer's Disease. With this training, they would know that watching TV is not the activity of choice. Many times they will fall asleep while watching TV. I know, this seems like a wonderful way for any care giver to get a little respite, but the sleep they get may interfere with their ability to sleep through the night, especially if that sleep period extends for several hours.

The use of mirrors can also create a problem. Remember, when we discussed the disease sufferer's regression? They may not recognize themselves in the mirror.

Let's assume the disease sufferer can find the bathroom and the mirror is on the wall opposite the door. They would attempt to enter the bathroom and seeing the unfamiliar face in the mirror, would apologize and close the door. They would believe the bathroom was occupied. This may be the cause of early incontinence. They found the bathroom, but couldn't wait for the occupant to leave. Sad, I know, but understandable. A woman is not as afraid of an unfamiliar face. They would be less disturbed, if they saw a stranger in the mirror. A woman usually smiles at another woman. Then of course, the reflection is smiling too. The family may see their disease suffer carrying on a conversation with their own reflection. Let's face it ladies, we would talk to a tree. It isn't hard to believe the disease sufferer would enjoy talking to the reflection in the mirror. The smile would be so disarming.

A gentleman on the other hand, would react quite differently. He would scowl at the reflection of another man in the mirror. A manly thing to do. The reflection would naturally scowl back, causing a threatening situation.

The male Alzheimer's Disease sufferer would perceive this as a threat and may attempt to fight the person he sees in his home. He may even search for a weapon to defend his home. A very dangerous time for the care giver.

Observe your disease sufferer for their reaction to their reflection in the mirror or glassed framed pictures for clues to explain aggressive behavior.

Many Alzheimer's Disease sufferers experience sun downing syndrome. It can be presented as agitated behavior or unexplained anxiety. It appears to be displayed as the day passes into night. Naturally, the person has become tired from the activities of the day and may even become frightened by the darkness. There may even be a reduction in their ability to perform tasks, as they show an increased confusion at this time, as well. A short nap at mid day may relieve this behavior. A calmer slower paced activity period, after about four o'clock, may reduce this reaction as well. Some disease sufferers need a small amount of medication to help them at this time of day. A need for intimacy may increase a male disease sufferer's desire for sex. Remember also, your male disease sufferer is regressing and sees himself as a much younger more sexually active man.

This behavior may become very aggressive and may need a physician's intervention as well. Don't be embarrassed to discuss this behavior with your physician.

Read on. The next chapter discusses many helpful interventions we developed through the years while observing our clients.

6

BEHAVIOR INTERVENTIONS
Life is a Dance

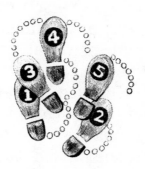

As I was traveling to one of my lectures, I heard a song that I thought was perfect for the care givers to hear.

Many times during the part of my lectures where I would discuss the behavior management interventions, I would notice that it seemed to disturb the participants. They would be shaking their heads and putting their hands up to gesture how simple the intervention was. I asked one of the participants what concerned him. He answered that the interventions were so simple he should have known what to do. I repeated what I had said earlier in my lecture. Until you understand what the disease is doing to the disease sufferer, one doesn't really know what to do. The behavior seems so bizarre.

This song, sung by John Michael Montgomery, was just perfect for the care givers in my audience. It was entitled, "Life's a Dance."

> *Life's a dance and you learn as you go*
> *Sometimes you lead and sometimes you follow*
> *Don't worry about what you don't know*
> *Cause life's a dance and you learn as you go.*

I have used this song verse to begin my lectures about behavior management interventions ever since. It instantly relieves the potential for guilty feelings, as I discuss interventions.

In Alzheimer's Disease, behavior can only be managed; it cannot be changed. We cannot stop the Alzheimer's disease sufferer from acting out. We can only redirect their attention and energy in a more purposeful direction.

In severe cases of aggressive, combative behaviors, anti-psychotic medications can be introduced. This intervention is not to eliminate the behavior management techniques, only to supplement them.

Depression, as mentioned in the previous chapters, can and often does coexist with the dementia. The use of an antidepressant many times lifts the depression, thereby improving the mood. The abilities to perform daily tasks and cognitive abilities frequently improve as well.

The level of deterioration can appear to improve; it actually does not. The existence of the depression had increased the difficulties of the Alzheimer's Disease sufferer.

Daily activities can help to control behavior and use up the extra energy the disease sufferer seems to have and allow them to tire enough for a good night's sleep.

Consistent Daily Schedule:

When the schedule of the Alzheimer's disease sufferer's day is dependable and the approaches by all the care givers are consistent, it gives the disease sufferer a sense of security. A world that their disease has turned upside down suddenly is less frightening and more dependable.

The schedule developed should be developed according to the dementia sufferer's personality and past activities.

For example, if the dementia sufferer took a bath every morning for 50 years, we should try to continue the pattern. If a person worked on the 11-7 shift the majority of their lives, we should not expect them to be able to sleep well during the night. Their body clock has already been set by their past experiences.

This is the very reason facilities specializing in dementia have activities and more staff on their 11-7 shifts than the traditional areas during the night to accommodate the residents who are wakeful during this time.

Allow short naps only, please. Care givers can unknowingly be the blame for sleepless nights.

If the dementia sufferers do not have activities to keep them occupied during the day, they may sleep away the day and be more wakeful at night. They may also become more restless and agitated, without something purposeful to do.

I know the stress of caring for this type of individual is extremely difficult, and when they sleep away the afternoon, it is often a welcomed relief for the care giver. This is an easy trap to fall into.

Early one morning, my then three-year-old son shook me awake. It really startled me. I told him it was only three o'clock in the morning and he should be asleep. He looked at me with his mischievous eyes, smiled and said "I used it all up!"

That's exactly what we are doing to the Alzheimer's Disease sufferer. We are using up all of their sleep during the day. Therefore, they are well rested and wandering throughout the night. The care giver does not get any sleep and the task of caring for their family member soon becomes exhausting.

This is a good time to bring up the need for help, since I am about to give you a few suggestions for behavior management activities. You don't have to do it alone. Consider hiring a little help.

The author of "When Love Gets Tough," Reverend Doug Manning, was lecturing about the importance of help with care giving. We are not all prepared to take on the care giving role, nor should we be. We all have limitations and should be honest about our ability to take on the care giving role. If you can't do it, get someone in who can. It is not a disgrace or a personal failure.

During the lecture, a young woman raised her hand. She said, "I have been crying for three weeks. When is it time to ask for help?" Reverend Manning answered, "When you have been crying for three weeks."

See, it's personal. Just know your limitations and be honest with yourself. It will keep you healthy and be much better for your family member. No one said you have to do it alone. We seem to tell ourselves that, especially the husbands. They somehow feel it is their responsibility and proves they love their spouse. Just try and remember the person before the disease took them away from you. Ask yourself if that person had expected you to become ill because you have taken on a task of caring for them all alone. Remember, if you exhaust yourself by taking on this extremely difficult task yourself, you will become ill and perhaps even have to be hospitalized. How do I know this, you ask? Statistics available through the Alzheimer's Association have proven time and time again that we lose the care givers much faster then we do the disease sufferers. Enough said?

Get help! No one will think the less of you:
When planning to hire a care giver to help you, which you will eventually need, make sure you discuss their training. They should have had at least a two-hour training course on Alzheimer's Disease for in-home care. They will know what is necessary and what approaches to use.

Now, let's continue with the suggestions for a daily schedule. Make sure you have a daily schedule to discuss with the care giver you hire, if one has been established. A history about your family members likes and dislikes is extremely helpful as well. Daily schedules should include usual times for meals, toileting schedules, if one has been identified, likes and dislikes for activities they may try, like reading, singing, taking walks, helping with chores and times for short naps. Your trained care giver can help you decide which activities your family may like. When your hired care giver is not there, the schedule established should be continued. It will keep the disease sufferer relaxed and calm, since their world is predictable and scheduled.

Don't get disappointed or jealous if the hired care giver is more successful then you were at getting the disease sufferer to comply. It happens all the time. Remember, the disease sufferer tries very hard to act correctly in public or around strangers. That is what is happening.

It is the same as our own children who seem to behave so much better for strangers than for their own parents. They know what they can get away with while we are there. They are not so sure of the strangers. There is also a significant reduction in anxiety for the hired care giver. They are not with the people 24-7 as you are. They are refreshed and rested.

By the way, family care giver, I used three shifts of care givers to care for my clients. You have been trying to do it alone.

Mealtime Suggestions:

The time that the Alzheimer's disease sufferer gets up and when they go to bed should remain the same. Meals should be on schedule as well. Snacks throughout the day can also help. It seems that if the person is well fed and rested, their behavior is more easily handled. Food should be offered in a manageable way, an egg sausage roll-up for breakfast perhaps. A grilled cheese sandwich and a cup of tomato soup, with a few pieces of peeled apple and a cup of milk for lunch is quite enough. Do not make the presentations of the meals too elaborate. Several types of glasses, all the flat wear and a center piece for the table are no longer necessary. It might be according to Emily Post but can be very confusing to the dementia sufferer. It's just too much to focus on.

Having snacks with extra fluids during the day can also help to keep the person's fluid consumption at a safe level.

The Alzheimer's Disease sufferer will not initiate the request for fluids, even though they may be very thirsty. They may not initiate feeding themselves either.

We had a lovely lady in our facility. She was the best example of a dignified lady of position who was used to entertaining. She was so personal and raised mealtime discussions to an art. She didn't, however, know how to start to eat. We simply filled her spoon, put it in her hand and helped her put it to her mouth. She would get the *ah ha* look on her face and was able to continue feeding herself, after we cued her or demonstrated for her that it was time to start eating now. Remember, hesitating to feed themselves doesn't always indicate that the person is not hungry. They may have forgotten how to start.

We also must allow the person to do whatever they can for themselves. It gives them a sense of accomplishment and maintains their dignity. Does it take longer? For sure! Can it be messier? You bet! But, please let them try by assisting them with cueing and demonstration, before you take the task away from them. The disease sufferers will get the unspoken message that they can't or that they are doing something wrong, if you take the ability away too early.

I suspected that for the sake of speed, some of my staff members were feeding a client I was sure could feed himself. The nurse aides assured me he couldn't feed himself any longer. He would keep his hands in his lap and allow them to feed him, but during crafts he would use his hands very well. He could sand wood and hammer with the best of his peers.

I showed them a little test. I put a cookie in his mouth. It stayed there for a few minutes and then began to sag due to the moisture. He instinctively raised his hands and caught it before it fell. Obviously, he had full use of his hands. He was just getting the message that he couldn't feed himself or that he was not doing it correctly, because the staff was doing it for him. Be careful of the silent messages you may be giving.

I looked at my staff and said, "He can feed himself, let him do it." With a little cueing, he was able to begin to feed himself again. Don't take-away abilities, since that only makes your own job more difficult.

Frequent snacks will not harm the person. They will actually help them to keep weight on. The latter stages of the disease will interfere with the absorption of nutrients. We have discussed that in previous chapters.

Please allow the person to help to prepare the meal or at least set the table or even fold the napkins. Being asked to participate in the activities during the day gives the person a feeling of self worth. They may not do it correctly, but please allow them the opportunity to try.

One daughter described her amazement at how the disease process affected her father's ability to make a simple sandwich. He made it inside out. He put mayonnaise on the slices of bread, put them together and piled the rest of the ingredients on top. He was quite proud of his accomplishment. His daughter did not comment and just let him do it himself. Maybe the next day she would ask him to set the table instead.

Personal Care:

Personal care can be one of the biggest challenges for the care giver, especially in the later stages of the disease process. The ability to preplan is essential. Remember, the disease sufferer thinks he is normal and can't imagine why someone is trying to give them a bath in the first place. Make sure you have all your supplies in the bathroom, before you bring in the disease sufferer. Allow the person to perform as much of the process as possible. Allowing them to hold a wash cloth makes it easier for you to complete the areas they cannot reach. If the bath cannot be accomplished, don't worry. Sitting on the toilet and receiving a sponge bath is quite acceptable. Don't use bath powder; it makes the bathroom floor dangerously slippery. Actually, bath powder can be very abrasive to the skin and may cause breakdown, if the person is incontinent. Toileting the disease suffer on a routine basis can prevent accidents and helps the disease sufferer maintain their dignity as well. Encourage the person to brush their own teeth and comb their own hair. Standing them in front of a mirror, while you stand beside them and demonstrate what you want them to do is very helpful. Remember the exercise group? An electric razor is safer than a razor, at this time.

Consistent and Patterned Activities:

If the activities experienced during the day are consistent, the dementia sufferer can be familiar with the pattern, not necessarily what is going to happen. Each day is a new day for them. That's why doing the same thing, every day, will not bother them. It can be quite boring for the care giver, but the benefits of a consistent schedule outweigh the boring times that may be experienced by the care givers.

One of our clients had gone out with their family for the afternoon. He became very anxious around three o'clock. He insisted on going back to the facility for the circle. The family asked about the circle, he mentioned, when they brought him back.

We explained that every day, at change of the shift, we brought our clients together, in a circle, to introduce them to the next shift. Now, these care givers were the same ones that worked last night but were new to our clients. There may have been a fill-in care giver at times. We would go around the circle and mention each resident name, greet them and try to compliment them on their hairdo or attire and introduce them to their care giver for the evening.

The response to this circle was amazing. As we went around the circle the residents awaiting their turn to be acknowledged actually looked forward to their turn. Do you wonder why?

We made them special, called them by name and relieved their anxiety by introducing them to their evening care givers. That is why the circle was so important to our residents.

We all need to be important and mean something to somebody. It was such an easy way to give our residents importance and peace of mind.

Introducing your family member to their care givers at home can have the same effect. A few compliments during the day can really make your family member feel important too.

Wherever the care giving is taking place, the rules remain the same: Dependable schedule and consistent predictable activities.

Daily Exercise:

If there is a walk, it should be at the same time every day. Exercise is an important component of the daily schedule. If you want to introduce physical activity along with a daily walk or if the person cannot walk for a long distance, try exercising to music.

Don't call it exercise. They won't want to come. Neither would you. Moving to music usually keeps their attention, but remember the therapist in the previous chapter. She had to demonstrate the movement herself. Your Alzheimer's Disease sufferer will be stronger and able to help with his care, and you will retain the strength to accomplish the tasks that you have. It is quite an enjoyable period of time and will lift the mood of the person and their care giver.

Music:

Music is very therapeutic, especially the songs that were popular when your family member was younger. Remember, they are going back in time. The songs of the big band era are very popular with the present generation of disease sufferers. The songs of the 50s and 60s will please the next generation of disease sufferers.

Let's pray they are fewer in number, due to research and development of miracle cures.

Religious songs are always popular. It brings to mind the strong faith that has been with the majority of sufferers most of their lives.

I particularly enjoy the old "Rock of Ages" type of song myself. I am catholic, and though our songs are beautiful, they do not seem to have the effect the old songs do. I think I am a closet Baptist. The old songs have words the disease sufferers remember. Some would sing them with tears in their eyes. Our group really loved the "Sing along with Mitch" songs. Easy to remember and fun to sing. My staff would complain that their friends would tease them when they would start singing these song at home.

They are the ones you can't get out of your head. The staff sang them so frequently, with our clients, they would sing them when they were with their friends as well.

Imagine, if you will, a group of about 10 Alzheimers' Disease clients belting out the song, "Show Me the Way to Go Home." The ladies would all giggle at the part, "I had a little drink about an hour ago and it went right to my head." What fun, we had. Simple huh?

Dinner out, anyone:

Feeling brave? Want to go out for dinner? Go right ahead, but use these tips. Preplan the place. Contact the restaurant in advance and advise them of your concerns. Select the menu in advance, as well. Request a table in a quiet area. With prior knowledge, the staff of your favorite restaurant can help you make the experience a pleasurable one for you and your disease sufferer. I discussed the lack of control in previous chapters. The switch that keeps us from insulting someone is not working for the Alzheimer's disease sufferer. Be prepared for embarrassing statements. If there is someone who looks differently, be assured that your disease sufferer will point that out for all to hear. "Boy, is she fat," may just pop out. Don't let this reaction ruin your adventure. If it does, then going out for dinner just isn't for you.

Vacations:

Vacations can still be enjoyed, as long as the change of scenery doesn't frighten the disease sufferer. That's when they may experience the catastrophic reactions we discussed earlier. They may become suddenly anxious and difficult to handle.

That doesn't mean you can't take a vacation. It is important for you to have a life as well.

I remember a young man who came to me for help. "I know my mom is lost to me and I will make sure that she is cared for. My father is well. He insists on caring for her himself. By doing so, he has taken himself away from me and my family as well. I have lost both my parents. I don't know how to help him."

I suggested he tell his father how he feels. He did so. His father didn't realize how his actions had affected the rest of the family. He visited with his sons family more often. They even took vacations together. While his mother spent time with care givers.

I always encouraged family members to take time for themselves, even if their disease sufferer couldn't go. They would all assure me they would. I suspected they may be telling me a fib, so I always requested pictures of their vacations. They had to be in the pictures.

Emergencies and hospitalization

Hospitalization of the Alzheimer's disease sufferer can be a traumatic experience for both themselves and their care givers.

Several pre-hospitalization steps can make a big difference.

1. Realize that there will have to be someone with the disease sufferer at all times. The hospitals cannot be there every minute. A familiar person is reassuring and calming. There are a few instances where the hospital will have personnel available to sit with your family member.

2. Discuss special needs with your physician, such as types of anesthesia, medications and additional support your family member may need.

3. Keep information about the disease sufferer handy just in case the hospitalization is for an emergency.

Several years ago a group of professionals and I set up a coalition, *Advocacy Coalition for the Cognitively Impaired* (ACCI). I know it is a long title, but it fit the situation and our purpose. We had all heard the sad stories from our family members, the acute care professionals and the emergency personnel about their disastrouss encounters with the Alzheimer's disease sufferer. We were attempting to create a form that would make immediate helpful information available.

They described aggression, combative behavior, elopement, and a total lack of understanding of the effect of hospitalization on an Alzheimer's disease sufferer.

We developed a form to accompany the patient that would be available to the hospital. I have included this form as the last page of the book. It describes the alzheimer disease sufferer's special needs and consideration. We actually were successful in getting one of our hospitals to make it a permanent part of their chart. That meant it would travel with the patient throughout their hospitalization.

The form is called, the Cognitively Impaired Alert. It contains all the information about how the patient reacts to their environment and the skills he or she still possesses, as well as the ones needing assistance. This is invaluable information for the healthcare workers who will minister to your family member.

Complete the form and make sure it is always available for emergency situations. The refrigerator door is an excellent place to put it. If you had an envelope with a magnet attached, you could keep other important information there as well, such as the doctor's name and phone number, list of present medications, both prescribed and over the counter, herbal supplements, allergies or sensitivities, pharmacy name and phone number, etc.

You are authorized to copy, modify or recreate the form, as needed. I would suggest that the form be copied on a machine capable of enlarging it to 8.5 X 11 inches.

All of these changes in behavior and your attempts to manage them can be very stressful.

The care giver must learn to recognize the symptoms of stress and remember to take time out themselves. The next chapter will discuss how to handle the stress experienced by the care givers , both family and professional. In the next chapter we will discuss a few easy ways to care for yourself.

Read on my friends.

7

STRESS MANAGEMENT
Care for The Care giver

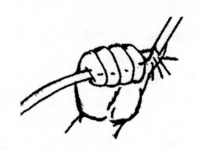

Everyone experiences stress in their daily lives, appointments to get to, children to get to school and through school. Trying to manage your responsibilities at home, as well as your own job, can also be a challenge.

Being a care giver, along with these other responsibilities, adds yet another dimension to the stress experienced in our daily lives.

In order to deal with the effects of stress, the body needs a little down time in between episodes. It needs to return to your baseline of normal functioning in order to recuperate.

When you add the care of an Alzheimer's Disease sufferer to the equation, the stress experienced does not allow for this down time. The care giver goes from the daily stressors to the extra stress of caring for their family member. This will eventually cause the care giver to break down, sometimes physically, sometimes mentally, sometimes both.

Many times, the care giver feels it is their responsibility to care for their family member and attempts to do it alone, be it a sense of guilt or loyalty that helped make that decision. Both can be destructive.

I have told many care givers that although you feel you can take care of your family member without help, you cannot. You cannot survive and you must, for the sake of your family.

We who are working in this field know we lose the care giver long before the Alzheimer's Disease sufferer.

Remember our discussion in the previous chapters? The Alzheimer's Disease sufferer does not realize the extent of his dementia or the problem it may be causing the family. They believe they are fine. This certainly reduces any stress for them but compounds the stress to their care giver.

For many years, I have taken care of the Alzheimer's Disease clients. I did it with three shifts of nurses, nurse aides and homemakers. These professional care givers had time away from the client to recuperate. Family care givers usually do not give themselves the luxury of that time away.

You must get help! There are many agencies out there that can help you. Financial agencies can handle your financial responsibilities, in order to allow you to have help at home or in a Specialized Care Unit, when the time comes.

Yes, I did say that placement in a Specialized Care Unit may be necessary.

The care giver, as well as the Alzheimer's Disease sufferer, deserves a decent quality of life.

Reverend Doug Manning has written a book entitled, "When Loves Gets Tough." He describes how when the care giver ignores their own life, as well as their continued involvement with the remainder of the family, there are many people imprisoned by this disease process instead of only one. The disease affects the entire family. You will need each other for support.

Remember the son I talked about earlier? He said his father chose to care for his mother alone. He knew his mother was lost to him. He loved her and wanted her to have the best of care, but because of his father's decision, he had lost both his parents, and his father was keeping his grandchildren from having a relationship with him as well as losing their grandmother.

Until this son told his father how he felt, the father had no idea how his actions were affecting the entire family. He was more receptive to suggestions of using professionals to help with his wife's care, after he and his son's conversation. It is a very difficult decision to make, but considering the care giver's quality of life as well, it is one that has to be made.

Reverend Manning says, "That's when love gets tough." He uses this statement in the beginning of his book. I suspect that was the inspiration for his choice of titles.

I was lucky enough to attend one of his lectures. While he was discussing the interventions for care and how professionals often had an easier time with the disease sufferer, due to their special training, a young woman raised her hand to ask a question.

"I have been crying for three weeks. When is it time to bring in professional help?" Reverend Manning's response seemed to put this all into perspective, "When you have been crying for three weeks," he said.

We are all different, with different strengths and weaknesses. Not all of us can or should handle the care of an Alzheimer's Disease sufferer.

As a nurse, I would probably be able to care for my husband for a while. On the other hand, my husband would be overwhelmed at the prospect of caring for me in the intimate way needed during this disease process. It is not because he loves me less than I love him? Not at all! We have discussed this type of situation at length, and we are comfortable with our own limitations.

Because you ask for help does not mean you have failed as a loving spouse or child. It simply means you realize the magnitude of the task, and you are willing to call in reinforcements.

Now, let's take a look at some signs of burnout and stress.

"At the Heart of Alzheimer's Disease," by Carol Simpson has outlined these signs and symptoms in a very understandable way. Read through them and be honest with yourself.

SIGNS OF BURNOUT

1. Are you curtailing visits and phone calls with close friends?
2. Have you given up activities that you have enjoyed for years?
3. Are you developing stress-related problems, such as back ache, headaches, chronic feelings of fatigue and depression?
4. Are you coming down with colds, flu and other illnesses more than usual?
5. Do you have a short temper? Do you get angry at the check out line at the grocery store? In traffic? With friends or family?

6. Do you have any outbursts at your loved one?
7. Have you gained or lost weight?
8. Do you have an unshakable feeling of despair or pessimism?
9. Are you crying? For no reason or over minor problems?
10. Do you complain about lack of sleep or chronic insomnia?
11. Do you have difficulty concentrating or performing familiar tasks?
12. Do you feel anxious about facing another day?

I told you in the very beginning about the incredible professionals I had the pleasure of meeting and learning from. Carol is certainly one of the professionals I spoke of. Did you answer the questions honestly? Doing so, may give you the insight into your own well being that many care givers fail to pursue.

There are physical, psychological and behavioral symptoms of stress. Here are just a few I received in a hand out from one of the many workshops I attended in my quest for knowledge about Alzheimer's Disease and its effect on the care giver. This particular one did not note an author that I could refer to.

PHYSICAL SYMPTOMS OF STRESS

Insomnia
Nightmares
Nausea or indigestion
Headaches or migraine's
Lower back pain
Eating too much
Dizziness
Over reliance on caffeine

Loss of appetite

Breathlessness
High Blood Pressure
Skin Rashes
Rapid Pounding Heartbeat
Allergies
Menstrual Irregularities
Loss of interest in sex
Use or abuse of
alcohol or other drugs
Impotence

PSYCHOLOGICAL SYMPTOMS OF STRESS

Feeling rushed
Under constant pressure

Feelings of isolation or loneliness

Catastrophic thinking

Difficulty making decisions

Feeling rejected
Feeling
misunderstood
Feeling vulnerable
to criticism
Difficulty asking
for help
Denial of problems

BEHAVIORAL SYMPTOMS OF STRESS

Deteriorating relationships
Withdrawal from others

Frequent arguments

Difficulty concentrating
Neglecting appearance
and hygiene
Frequent forgetting of
information

Any of these symptoms sound familiar? Don't worry; you're not alone. We have all been there. The problem is recognizing them and taking action to keep yourself healthy.

Remember! You're important too.

The Alzheimer's Association frequently publishes topical information. Here is an example of one of those helpful publications.

CARING FOR THE CARE GIVER

1. Become Educated
2. Know what resources are available: Day Care, meals on wheels, support groups and the Alzheimer's Association.
3. Have a Daily Schedule but be flexible.
4. Legal and Financial Planning: Durable Power of Attorney, living wills, future medical care, housing.
5. Get help: family, friends, community resources
6. Take Care of Yourself! : Nutrition, diet, exercise
7. Give yourself Credit: You are not a super person. Take one day at a time.

All of these suggestions are useful and possible. Give yourself a gift and use them. We've started the first one together. We will be discussing the community resources in the final chapter. We have already discussed the need for a daily schedule for the Alzheimer's Disease sufferer. Remember to be flexible.

Getting legal and financial help is essential. There will be a listing of resources in this area in the final chapter as well.

I will repeat the last two sentences for emphasis. Take care of yourself, and remember to give yourself credit. Few people could do what you are attempting to do, but remember you are not a super person.

Take one day at a time reminds me of my work with cancer patients. Their group was called, "One Day at A Time." It is interesting how these two diseases parallel. Both are devastating and both are frustrating, because at some point there is nothing else you can do.

That is why it is so important for the care givers to get help and support. The support groups offered by the Alzheimer's Association can be very helpful.

Don't be afraid or ashamed to reach out for help. The support groups are care givers like you who come together to discuss problems and share solutions. They are the ones who understand and will listen. As a care giver, you do have rights, you know. We all pay more attention to the ill family member than we do the person who has become responsible for their care. James Kenney and Stephen Spicer, who wrote "Caring For Your Aging Parent-A Practical Guide to the Challenges; The Choices," felt that the care givers needed their own bill of rights. The following is the result of their efforts.

CARE GIVER'S BILL OF RIGHTS

- You must survive and you have that right!
- Sometimes you need a few hours away from your elderly or impaired parent or spouse.
- You have the right to go off and find yourself again in some personal pursuit.
- You have the right to get help. You are not indispensable - others can act in your place.

- You have the right to be patient with yourself and your aging or impaired parent or spouse; it is even more important to be patient with yourself.

Now that we have given you permission to ask for help. Here are a few suggestions:

Make a list of jobs that need to be done. Good! Now hand them out to family and friends. Go out and play a round of golf, or out to lunch with friends. How about taking a trip? No, that is not being selfish. This is taking care of you.

Now that you know there are services available, learn to use them. It will keep you healthy and strong and more able to continue caring for your loved one.

Friends, you can help too. Offer to do errands. Stay in contact. Your friend needs your support. Listen. It is so important for the care giver to have someone familiar to talk to. Offer to bring over a meal. Better yet, if you are comfortable enough, offer to spend a few hours with the disease sufferer so their care giver can have a much needed break.

Caring for yourself is important. Let your friends and family help. Your survival is important to them, as well as to your Alzheimers' Disease sufferer.

8

GRIEVING PROCESS
The forgotten step

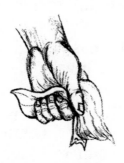

The Alzheimer's Disease Association refers to the Alzheimer's Disease process as the never ending funeral. The family members are usually dealing with the disease for at least ten years after it is diagnosed. They have explained to me many times how difficult it is to grieve a living person but grieve they must.

Grief, as explained by Elizabeth Koebler Ross is a process comprised of specific steps. One goes through these steps at there own pace. The steps she describes are:

- Anger
- Denial
- Bargaining
- Acceptance

A seemingly simple process to follow, if one was not dealing with a disease like Alzheimers. This disease process doesn't follow the rules. It continues to throw the family back to the first step with each loss.

As mentioned in the previous chapter, support group meetings with other care givers can be a god-send for the family care givers.

Early stage Alzheimer's Disease support groups are also available for the disease suffer. There they will learn about the techniques they can use to support their failing memories. Written notes, labeling drawers and cabinets, etc. Discussing their feelings and fears to fellow sufferers can be invaluable at this time, as well. These support groups usually meet at the same time in the same building, but in separate rooms.

Lets take a look at why this grief process is difficult to follow for the Alzheimers' Disease sufferer and their families.

With the horror and profound grief experienced with the initial diagnosis certainly comes anger. "Why me?" "Why us?" Denial, surely. "This just can't be true. We need a second opinion, a third opinion. Please someone, tell me this isn't true."I certainly agree with the second and perhaps third opinion, especially considering the other possibilities for the symptoms of memory loss, confusion and personality changes discussed in the first few chapters of this book.

Anger about the situation and sometimes anger directed at the disease sufferer is the most troubling reaction they experience attempting to deal with this disease process. "Why me? I was looking forward to a happy relaxed retirement, now this." This reaction, as described by Koebler-Ross, is normal. You are not a terrible, unfaithful, selfish spouse or child for experiencing this anger. You know or will shortly find out how difficult dealing with this can be. That is why you must learn to accept help. A bit of a reminder from the previous chapter.

Grief counseling can be very helpful at this time, but unfortunately very few family care givers seek this type of therapy to help them deal with this dreaded disease. "How can I grieve a person who is standing in front of me?" I hope after reading this chapter you will be able to. Grief counseling can help you deal with your feelings, which will ultimately enable you to better care for your Alzheimers' Disease suffer and care for yourself at the same time.

During one of these counseling sessions, a young girl began to sob uncontrollably. When asked by the facilitator what had caused her reaction, she said it was her guilt. She felt she must be a terrible daughter, because she had wished her father dead rather than see him suffer through this dreaded disease process. "What a terrible child she must be." Not at all. She simply wanted to spare her father the years of suffering he was facing. Bargaining.

Although my father didn't die of Alzheimers' Disease, I was attending this grief counseling support group. I had set it up for our facility support group families. I was surprised at my reaction. I had expected to remain detached during this session, as I did not have anyone in my family suffering with Alzheimers' Disease. How wrong I was.

My father died at 58 years of age, and apparently I hadn't dealt with my anger either. I was really mad at God. I am a religious person and always tried to accept what I was expected to deal with in life. My father's death changed all that. I found myself explaining to the group the meeting I was going to have with God, when and if I ever meet him, about how unfair I thought my father's death was. I described to them the bargaining I did as my father was slipping away. "Please!, Please!

give me half of his illness so that he can survive a little longer," I pleaded. Since I was married with a small child, I didn't think it was right to take his place, but I was willing to shorten my life to save his. Interestingly enough, he had gone through his grief process and was at the acceptance stage. His three daughters and his loving wife, however, were not as lucky. We hadn't arrived at the level of peace he experienced at the end of his life. You see? We are all the same, aren't we?

Acceptance seems to be the most illusive step in this grieving process. Just as the family members and the newly diagnosed disease sufferers come to terms with the situation they find themselves in, the disease process throws them a curve ball. The situation changes. There is further regression, further loss of abilities and more confusion.

The process begins again. The only merciful element in the disease process is that the disease sufferer eventually becomes unaware of his decline in abilities and loss of function. There is a considerable decline in their anxiety. Especially if their care givers have learned the nuances of handling the disease sufferer. The care givers, however, remain all too aware of the continued decline. This situation increases their anxiety and stress. More grief for the new loss of function and their loss of freedom from this disease process. Stress, if not addressed, will lead to illness. We lose many of our care givers long before the Alzheimers' Disease sufferers.

Not everyone is expected to be able to deal with this disease process. You must be honest with yourself . You are not a terrible person or an unloving spouse simply because you need help and support. As I mentioned in a previous chapter, I use three shifts of nurses to do what most family care givers are attempting to do alone. Please allow yourself to grieve and accept help.

There are amazing professionals out there waiting to help you. Accepting their help does not make you a failure. I refer to the next chapter as the lifeboat. We, the professional care givers in your community, have created a life boat of services for you. You simply need to allow yourself to get in.

9

COMMUNITY RESOURCES
The life boat

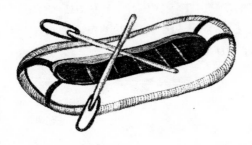

You have already used one of the most important resources available to you, education. The remainder of the resources come together to create the "lifeboat" you will need to survive.

Attending Support Group meetings should be the next thing on your list. The level and the amount of community resources you may need to help you care for the Alzheimer's Disease sufferer depends upon the stage they are in.

Financial and legal arrangements are important to take care of in the early stages. The judgement of the early stage Alzheimer's Disease sufferer is impaired. They can be swindled easily. Having someone appointed to handle their financial affairs is essential. It can be quite a challenge convincing the disease sufferer of this however. Remember, this stage is when paranoia is a problem. They may think you are trying to steal their money. Do not be offended. This is not personal. It can be a family member or a Trust Officer who is appointed to handle their financial affairs. If there is no one to assume the responsibility for the disease sufferer, a Guardian may have to be appointed to assure their safety.

Make sure the disease sufferer's wishes will be followed, if there is an emergency. What do they want done? An Elder Law Attorney can be extremely helpful at this time. Having these wishes in writing in the home is vital.

In the earlier stages, having someone checking on them frequently and perhaps having meals delivered may be sufficient. If family is near-by, preparing meals and labeling them can help the disease sufferer remember to eat. Members of your church are a great source to tap for help. A visit by a member of the disease sufferers church can be just the person to check in on them while they are still able to remain at home.

Placing labels on cabinets to locate items and having a large calendar to remind them of appointments and speed dial for family and emergency numbers can be really helpful.

As the disease progresses, the ability to make safe decisions is impaired. A son who lived out of town was concerned about his mother's safety. She would not permit anyone who appeared medical to enter her home. Describing the care giver as a personal secretary allowed his mother to maintain her dignity and still allow protection in her home. It even gave her something to brag about to the girls in her bridge club.

The level of care needed and what family members are available for care may effect the decision to allow the disease sufferer to stay in their own home. Remember, not everyone can or should assume the care of an Alzheimer Disease sufferer. The level of care that can be accomplished by professional care givers at home will naturally depend on the financial resources available.

Investigating existing insurances policies and what they will pay for is vital. Many Long-Term Care Insurance policies will address the private duty care of the insured at home. Or perhaps an Assisted Living Facility will be more appropriate. Many insurance policies can also help with these expenses as well.

When the disease reaches the middle to late stages, a Specialized Care Unit may be the best place for your disease sufferer. Yes, I did have the nerve to suggest that professionals may just be better equipped to handle the disease sufferer at this point than the family can.

The family can certainly assume this care throughout the disease process as long as they remember that everyone in the family deserves a good quality of life, not only the disease sufferer. Remember the Care Givers Bill of Rights? You must survive, and you have that right.

The Alzheimer's Association in your area will have a list of legal services, facilities and professionals who can provide services to the Alzheimer's Disease sufferer and their families. The information families can receive from the Alzheimer Association is invaluable and spans all aspects of concern, including legal and ethical issues. The following information will be very helpful to the families of the Alzheimer's disease sufferer.

LEGAL AND ETHICAL ISSUES:

Although Alzheimer's disease is primarily a medical problem, caring for the person with Alzheimer's disease has a great deal to do with the law. Laws vary from state to state and are changing frequently, usually in response to the needs of an increasingly larger and better organized population.

Elder Law is the name given to the field that deals with the issues of aging, incapacity, long term care planning, government benefits programs, protective services, guardianship and tax and estate planning. Elder law attorneys do estate planning and prepare living wills and durable power of attorney. They can help to explain the complex issues of Medicare, Medicaid and public benefits. We, in the field of Alzheimer's disease care, feel the person with Alzeimer's disease should maintain their freedom to make choices for as long as possible. We believe the person should be able to make their own decisions about their own affairs for as long as they can. The following issues should be considered:

FREEDOM TO MAKE CHOICES:

Does the person have the ability to make sound decisions - the physician, working with a lawyer, social worker and the Alzheimer's disease victim's family can help make this evaluation. Is the person aware of his condition? If people are unaware of their medical condition or if they do not understand the nature of their medical condition, they may be reluctant to plan anything.

RESPECT FOR INDIVIDUAL RIGHTS:

Recognize the right of the Alzheimer's disease sufferer to make his own decisions. Identify services available to assist the family and disease victim to make legal and financial decisions. Identify the options available for managing the financial and medical decisions.

ETHICAL ISSUES:

Even though there is a loving family attempting to make the decisions for the Alzheimer's disease victim, protests may still be heard from the person, their spouse or other family members. Legal and ethical conflicts may arise such as, what does the person want or who would the person choose for a spokesperson, when communication is no longer possible, to make decisions concerning financial and healthcare decisions? Can the interests of the Alzheimer's disease victim and his family be fairly represented?

FINANCIAL MANAGEMENT:

It is important to set up a system to manage the person's financial affairs, if the time comes when they cannot act on their own. In the case of the Alzheimer's disease sufferer, it *is* when they cannot act on their own.

TRUST OFFICER:

A trust officer not only manages the financial interests of their client, many times they also manage the health care needs. They work closely with the agencies in their area to bring the necessary care to their client at the most reasonable cost. Their task, and it can be a daunting one, is to make sure their client will have enough money left to receive the level of care they need.

FINANCIAL PLANNER:

A financial planner can help individuals set up a system to manage their financial affairs. It is never too soon to investigate this type of professional consultation. Health care costs continue to rise. We should be prepared for the eventuality that we or our loved ones may have costly health care needs as we age.

GERIATRIC CARE MANAGERS:

This person would be able to assist the family in managing the medical care that the disease sufferer may need. They would be the one setting up the care needed and monitoring its effectiveness. This service is especially valuable if the family is not living close by.

GUARDIANS:

Guardians would be in place for the persons who could no longer handle their affairs and there is no property management system in place. It would be necessary to apply to the state court to have a guardian appointed. This would only be necessary if a trust officer or a person with the power of attorney to act for the person has not been named.

FINANCIAL TOOLS

DURABLE POWER OF ATTORNEY:

A power of attorney is a written delegation of authority to another person or persons to act as "agent" of the incapacitated person when assistance of another person is needed. It is important to have the wording in the document say that it is valid even if disability occurs.

LIVING TRUSTS:

A trust is a contract between a person who owns property, sometimes called the grantor, and a person selected to manage that property, called the trustee.

JOINT BANK ACCOUNTS:

A joint bank account can be managed by either Co-owner and either is able to manage the account.

IN-HOME CARE

PRIVATELY HIRED CARE GIVERS:

Care givers may be hired by the family. The family becomes responsible for determining if this person is capable of caring for their family member. If the private care giver does not handle their own finances, the family or client is responsible for this activity (i.e., payroll taxes, Workers' Compensation , disability insurance.)

COMPANIONS:

This is an individual who could monitor the client, remind them to take their medications, do light housekeeping, prepare meals and take the client to Dr's appointments and do the grocery shopping. This type of care is not hands on care. If the disease sufferer needs to be dressed, bathed or assisted with toileting, this level of care is no longer appropriate. At this level, the care giver is not trained to perform personal care.

HOME HEALTH AIDE/ CERTIFIED NURSE AIDES:

A Home Health aide can perform all the tasks of the Companion, along with any physical care that may be necessary. They may also, if trained, assist the person with their medications. They cannot, however, dispense these medications. A licensed nurse must dispense medications (place medications in daily or weekly containers), etc. They may not administer medications or administer treatments. There are machines that can dispense daily medications, but it would still be necessary for a licensed nurse to set up these machines.

LICENSED PRACTICAL NURSE / REGISTERED NURSE:

If the disease sufferer can no longer take their medications with some assist and reminding, then a licensed nurse must administer them. If there are treatments ordered for the disease sufferer such as insulin injections, wound care, naso-gastric or gastric feedings, a licensed individual must perform these treatments. If a family member has been trained by a professional, they can also perform these tasks.

LICENSED PRIVATE DUTY HOME HEALTH AGENCY:

A licensed private duty home health agency can care for the disease sufferer from 1 to 24 hours according to the persons needs or the family wishes. They employ companions, home health aides, certified nurse aides and licensed nurses. Payment for this level of care is on an hourly basis. The care is paid for by the client or their family, trust account, some private insurances, long term care insurance, worker's compensation and veterans' administration benefits.

LICENSED MEDICARE HOME HEALTH AGENCY:

Medicare will pay for care in the home on an intermittent basis and if ordered by a physician. A person can receive medicare home health care after hospitalization and without hospitalization, if the person's needs meet the criteria for this type of care and he has a physician's order for the care.

Medicare home health can access personal care, physical therapy, occupational therapy, speech therapy and social services

HOSPICE:

Hospice will come into place in the last stages of the disease process. It will allow the person to remain at home until their death. It is palliative care. This means they will be there to see that the disease sufferer is comfortable, well cared for and as free of pain as possible, until the end of their life.

Hospice will also be able to provide the equipment needed by this level of care (hospital bed, wheel chair, etc.)

CARE OPTIONS

ADULT DAY SERVICES:

There are several agencies that offer Adult Day Services. They are a Godsend for the caregiver. They allow a few hours away from the impaired person for respite.

Interestingly enough, it is quite difficult to convince the caregivers they should allow themselves a little free time.

Many Adult Day Services provide what they call *scholarships* to assist the families with this type of care.

SAFE RETURN:

While the Alzheimer's Disease sufferer is still at home, you should seriously consider enrolling them in the Safe Return program offered by the Alzheimer's Association. It is a national program that will be able to locate your family member should they wander away from home. The caregiver should also be enrolled, to assure that care can continue in an emergency.

MEDICAL ALARM SYSTEM:

A medical alarm system is another consideration. They are becoming quite popular and will provide an additional degree of security to the family of the disease sufferer. If an accident occurs in the home, help is at hand immediately to address your needs.

HOME CARE PHYSICIANS:

Yes, believe it or not, Home Care Physicians are becoming the new trend. This is an incredible service for the caregivers of the Alzheimer's disease sufferer. The preparation for and going to the doctor's office can often be very traumatic for the disease sufferer and their caregiver. Many physicians have begun offering home visits for these situations.

PAYMENT SOURCES

PRIVATE PAY:

The responsibility of the disease sufferer or their family.

MEDICARE INSURANCE:

Would pay for intermittant care at home and skilled care as ordered by a physician.

LONG TERM CARE INSURANCE:

Long term care insurance will pay for home care and facility care, according to the program the person has selected.

MEDICAID:

Medicaid is a medical assistance program jointly financed by state and federal governments for low income individuals. The person needing assistance will have to apply for this assistance and will be evaluated according to their care needs and financial ability to pay for this care.

VA HEALTHCARE, PENSIONS & BURIAL BENEFITS

Unfortunately, many families overlook the Department of Veterans Affairs when searching for agencies to help with the costs of care for Alzheimer's disease sufferers.

In an article written by the Department of Veterans Affairs, they explain the services available.

The benefits they offer include, but are not limited to; service connected disability compensation, non-service connected disability pensions, assistance with nursing homes, assisted living facilities and home health care, medical treatment, prescription drugs, and reimbursement for the cost of adapting a home or a motor vehicle due to a veteran's service- connected disability.

You might be unaware of the benefits available if you are a veteran, or the surviving spouse of a veteran. There is a wide assortment of benefits that vary depending on income, wartime service, whether a veteran has a service-connected disability and the type of discharge the veteran received. They offer assistance with these benefits and with determining eligibility criteria, and it is only a phone call away.

TYPES OF FACILITIES

ASSISTED LIVING FACILITY:

In the early stages of the disease process, the disease sufferer's needs can easily be met in this type of facility. The disease sufferer will have staff observing them. but they would be able to be somewhat independent. This type of facility would not be appropriate for a wanderer or a disease sufferer with complicated behavior management concerns.

SPECIALIZED ALZHEIMER'S AND RELATED DISEASE UNIT:

An environment set up especially to meet the needs of the Alzheimer's and related dementia clients. The difference is immediately noticeable. There are organized activities throughout the day and early evening hours. They are secured so it would be appropriate for the wandering client. The activities also help to manage the difficult behaviors associated with this disease process. The staffing is at a higher level in speciality units. The staff has been trained to understand and care for the dementia client.

LONG TERM CARE/REHABILITATION FACILITY:

In the later stages of the disease process, the care that is necessary increases. That care is better provided in a skilled facility. The need to protect the client from wandering and the need for activities to manage behavior are no longer necessary. The care is now primarily physical and the client is usually incontinent and having difficulty eating. As the Alzheimer's disease sufferer is mercifully coming to the end of their life we cannot forget the family and the care givers. They will continue to suffer the loss of their loved one or, as bazaar as it might sound, feel guilty about the feelings of relief that they may be experiencing.

Remember the ability to mourn for this person has been put on the back burner, due to the overwhelming experience of caring for the Alzheimer's disease sufferer. The caregivers, and especially the spouse, are extremely vulnerable at this time for depression due to the loss of their spouse and also for the loss of their purpose in life. Many times, these caregivers have not had the time to develop other interests. Their entire focus has been on caring for the disease suffer, and now he is gone. What now? The family and spouse of the Alzheimer's disease sufferer will continue to need their friends around them at this sad time in their lives. Thank you to all the friends who have remained in contact with the families during the course of their loved one's disease process. Please remain close by for a while yet. They still need your love and support.

I usually closed my lectures with yet another poem I have had for many years:

THE JOY OF LIVING

If nobody smiled, and nobody cheered,
and nobody helped us along;
If each one only looked after himself,
and the good things all went to the strong;

If nobody cared just a little for you,
and nobody cared for me,
And we all stood alone in the battle of life,
what a dreary world this would be!

Life is sweet because of the friends we have made
and the things which in common we share.
We want to live on, not because of ourselves,
but because of the people who care.

It's giving and doing for somebody else -
it's on that all life's splendor depends.
The joy of this world when we summed it all up
is found in the making of FRIENDS...

I know we have made more friends for the Alzheimer's disease sufferers because you have read this book up to this point. I hope I have helped the Alzheimer's disease care givers better understand the disease sufferer and to know they are not trying to cause a problem for you. It this dreaded disease that is causing them to behave in such a troubling way. For those who read this book so they can better understand Alzheimer's disease and the behaviors it causes, THANK YOU! I now know that anyone you may meet in the future who might be suffering with Alzheimer's Disease or caring for victims of this terrible disease now have a few more FRIENDS to call on for help and support. I certainly hope I have made a few friends and that this book has relieved some of the anguish suffered by the Alzheimer's disease sufferer and their families.

In the last section of this book, I have included website addresses and telephone numbers of the Agencies and Associations referred to in this chapter.

God Bless you all,

Sandy

RESOURCES AVAILABLE

Alzheimer's Association National Office
Provides information about Alzheimer's Disease, resources, research advances, publications and events.
225N. Michigan Avenue, Fl. 17
Chicago, IL 60601
1-800-272-3900
www.alz.org

Alzheimer's Association Houston & Southeast Texas Chapter
2242Holcombe Blvd.
Houston, Texas 77030
1-713-266-6400

Alzheimer's Association Florida Gulf Coast Chapter
Sarasota/Manatee
1230 South Tuttle Avenue
Sarasota, Fl 34239
1-941-365-8883

Medicaid
Medicaid is a medical assistance program jointly funded by state and federal governments for low income individuals.
www.cms.hhs.gov/home/medicaid.asp
www.myflorida.com/accessflorida
1-866-762-2237/1-866-76-ACCES[S]

US Dept of Veterans Affairs
www.gibill.va.gov/
VA Benefits - 1-800-827-1000
Health Care Benefits - 1-877-222-8387

Sarasota County Veterans Service Office*
Sarasota, Fl. - 1-941-861-2899
tacton@scgov.net

Long Term Care Insurance
42 Ladd Street 2nd Floor
East Greenwich, RI 02816
www.LTCinsurance.com

American Association of Long Term Care Insurance
www.aaltc.org

US National Institute of Health, National Institute on Aging Alzheimer's Disease Education & Referral Center (ADEAR)
P.O. Box 8250
Silver Springs MD 209-8250
www.alzheimers.nia.nih.gov

Eldercare Locator 1-800-677-1116
This service of the Administration on Aging, funded by the Federal Government, provides information and referrals to respite care and other home and community services offered by state and Area Agencies on Aging.
www.eldercare.gov

National Academy of Elder Law Attorney
NAELA defines the scope of elder law and gives the latest news about legal issues affecting the elderly. Includes a searchable directory.
www.naela.org

Florida Geriatric Care Managers Association, Inc.
FGCMA (A Chapter of the National Association of Professional Care Managers)
9715 West Broward Blvd. PMB 206
Plantation, Florida 33321
www.fgcma.org

Local Veteran Services are listed under County Services in your telephone book.

THE AUTHOR

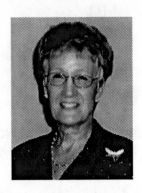

Sandy Kehoe was born and raised in Downingtown, Pennsylvania, which is just west of Philadelphia. She began her career in Acute Care Nursing in a 265 bed hospital and eventually became the Risk Manager for that same hospital.

She moved to Houston, Texas where she worked extensively; educating the community about the Alzheimer's disease process and the resources available and helping companies develop the specialized Alzheimer's environments. She later moved to Florida, accepting a position as Administrator of an Assisted Living facility.

Sandy has worked in several areas of the health care field giving her a broad perspective of the services available for the Alzheimer Disease sufferer. She is presently the Administrator of a Licensed Private Duty agency serving Sarasota and surrounding areas.

As a registered nurse with an Associate degree in the Applied Science of Nursing, community education continues to be the most important aspect of her nursing practice.

For the past eleven years, Sandy has lived in Sarasota, Florida with Jim, her husband of forty years. Her son Michael and his wife Susan also reside in Sarasota.

COGNITIVELY IMPAIRED ALERT

This form is to be part of medical record

Name: _____
Date assessed: _____
Name client prefers to be called: _____
Conversational interests: _____
Former occupation: _____
Favorite foods: _____
Cultural or religious preferences: _____
Form completed by: _____
Facility: _____
Phone: _____
Physician: _____
Contact person: _____
Phone: _____

Photo

CIRCLE OR CHECK ALL THAT APPLY

BEHAVIOR

1. Agitated   2. Quarrelsome   3. Affectionate
4. Depressed   5. Cooperative   6. Disruptive
7. Withdrawn   8. Suspicious   9. Flirtatious
10. Verbally aggressive   11. Paces
12. Physically aggressive   13. Wanders
14. Removes clothing   15. Sense of humor
16. Sees/hears things not there
17. Reliable with what he/she says

HELPFUL TIPS

_____
_____
_____
_____
_____
_____
_____
_____

COMMUNICATION

1. Preferred language
2. Has difficulty understanding words   [Yes] [No]
3. Has difficulty expressing words   [Yes] [No]
4. Communicates using_____
5. Level of compression   [High] [Moderate] [Low]

DRESSING

1. Needs assistance with _____
2. Must be dressed   [Yes] [No]

HEARING

1. Good   [Yes] [No]
2. Impaired   [Yes] L_____ R_____ [No]
3. Deaf   [Yes] L_____ R_____ [No]
4. Hearing Aid   [Yes] L_____ R_____ [No]

SIGHT

1. Good   [Yes] [No]
2. Limited   [Yes] L_____ R_____ [No]
3. Blind   [Yes] L_____ R_____ [No]
   Wears glasses   [Yes] [No]

NUTRITION

1. Feed self / Minor assistance / Total assistance
2. Right handed _____ Left handed _____
3. Regular diet_____ Cut foods _____
   Finger foods_____ Pureed foods_____
4. Special diet?_____
5. Dentures   [Yes] U_____ L_____ [No]

TOILETING

1. Continent   [Yes] [No]
2. Incontinent bladder _____ bowel _____
3. Incontinent products   [Yes] [No]
4. Take to bathroom every two hours   [Yes] [No]

TRANSFER

1. Independent   [Yes] [No]
2. Walks with supervision   [Yes] [No]
3. Walks with assistive device   [Yes] [No]
   Cane_____ Walker_____ Wheelchair_____
4. Bed to chair with assist   [Yes] [No]
5. Total bed rest   [Yes] [No]

SAFETY

1. Can use call light   [Yes] [No]
2. Can express discomfort   [Yes] [No]
3. Sundowners   [Yes] [No]

BATHING

1. Level of assistance   [Low] [Medium] [High]
2. Must be bathed   [Yes] [No]

COMMUNICATION TECHNIQUES

SMILE! APPROACH SLOWLY! MAKE EYE CONTACT! INTRODUCE YOURSELF EACH TIME YOU APPROACH.
EXPLAIN ALL PROCEDURES BEFORE YOU ATTEMPT THEM! SPEAK SLOWLY & SOFTLY.
USE SIMPLE SENTENCES TO GIVE INFORMATION. WAIT FOR A RESPONSE.
IF NO RESPONSE, REPEAT EXACTLY!